Essentials of Allergy

D1330175

M Thirumala Krishna PhD MRCP(UK) DNB
Specialist Registrar in Allergy and Clinical Immunology,
and Honorary Clinical Lecturer, Southampton General
Hospital and University of Southampton, Southampton,
UK

George Mavroleon PhD
Specialist in Allergy, 10–12 Sfakion Street, Chania,
73134 Crete, Greece

Stephen T Holgate MD DSc FRCP
MRC Clinical Professor of Immunopharmacology,
and Honorary Consultant Physician, University of
Southampton and Southampton General Hospital,
Southampton, UK

with a Foreword by Professor Stephen R Durham MA MD FRCP,
Professor of Allergy and Respiratory Medicine,
National Heart & Lung Institute, London, UK

MARTIN DUNITZ

© 2001 Martin Dunitz Ltd, a member of the Taylor and Francis group

First published in the United Kingdom in 2001 by
Martin Dunitz Ltd
The Livery House
7–9 Pratt Street
London NW1 0AE

Tel: +44-(0)20-7482-2202
Fax: +44-(0)20-7267-0159
E-mail: info.dunitz@tandf.co.uk
Website: http://www.dunitz.co.uk

A CIP catalogue for this book is available from the British Library

ISBN 1-85317-783-0

Distributed in the United States by:
Blackwell Science Inc.
Commerce Place, 350 Main Street
Malden MA 02148, USA
Tel: 1-800-215-1000

Distributed in Canada by:
Login Brothers Book Company
324 Salteaux Crescent
Winnipeg, Manitoba R3J 3T2
Canada
Tel: 1-204-224-4068

Distributed in Brazil by:
Ernesto Reichmann Distribuidora de Livros, Ltda
Rua Coronel Marques 335, Tatuape 03440-000
Sao Paulo
Brazil

Composition by Wearset, Boldon, Tyne and Wear
Printed and bound in Italy by Printer Trento

Contents

Foreword

Atopy, a predisposition to IgE-mediated allergic disorders, is defined as the presence of a positive skin test and/or raised serum allergen-specific IgE to one or more common inhaled allergens. Atopy affects some 30–40 per cent of the population of westernised countries. Approximately half these individuals develop clinically significant allergic disorders, which include allergic rhinitis, conjunctivitis and bronchial asthma. Allergic rhinitis is particularly common and, although often trivialized, may have a major impact on quality of life with impaired performance at work/school, poor sleep quality and interference with leisure pursuits. Less common but potentially life-threatening conditions include anaphylaxis to certain foods and to the venom of stinging insects.

Essentials of Allergy covers the diagnosis and clinical management of the common allergies. The less common eosinophilic lung diseases and extrinsic allergic alveolitis are also expertly covered. The text is easy to read and complemented by the many tables and illustrations. The diagnostic algorithms and detailed information on drugs and doses are particularly helpful. Frequently, allergic disorders coexist. Whereas the first port of call for patients with multiple allergies is, quite rightly, the general practitioner, such patients may benefit from the multidisciplinary approach offered by an allergy specialist. In this sense, *Essentials of Allergy* 'fills the gap' by providing a timely and comprehensive account of the common allergic disorders. The book should be of particular interest to general practitioners, nurses and organ-based specialists and will be a valuable teaching aid for allergists.

Professor Stephen R Durham
Professor of Allergy and Respiratory
Medicine
Upper Respiratory Medicine
National Heart & Lung Institute
London

Preface

Most medical specialties are focused on specific organs, while others, such as immunology, cover a series of interdependent events relating to the host and its ability to protect itself against the environment. The practice of allergy falls somewhere between the two: strong organ-based expression (e.g. asthma, atopic eczema) but often extending to other systems. The definition of 'allergy' also leads to confusion – on the one hand, meaning a group of hypersensitivity disorders with well-defined immunological mechanisms and, on the other, covering a range of intolerances to various environmental factors for which clear mechanisms have not been defined.

Different health systems provide services to allergy patients through both the primary and secondary care sectors, with large variations between countries. Because of the high prevalence of allergic disease, its rising trend over time and the appearance of new allergens to which patients react, we felt there was a need for an easily digestible text on the subject, which was highly accessible to those wishing to obtain a good background relatively easily. We have targeted the book towards both primary and secondary health care. The text is divided into 13 chapters covering different aspects of hypersensitivity responses. Thus, the book is clinically oriented and should be valuable to trainees in allergy, respiratory medicine and general (internal) medicine, as well as to general practitioners and the professions allied to medicine.

There is a pressing need to improve the quality of care that patients with allergic disease receive. It is with this in mind that we hope that this text provides a useful and accessible source of practical information.

M Thirumala Krishna
George Mavroleon
Stephen T Holgate

Diagnostic tests in allergy

Introduction

Although there is no substitute for a good history in clinical medicine, laboratory tests are often required to strengthen the clinical diagnosis and to provide a means of, objectively, evaluating the disease, its severity and its response to treatment. This chapter focuses on various *in vivo* and *in vitro* tests employed in the investigation and diagnosis of allergic disease. Some of these tests are used mostly as research tools but, nevertheless, they provide useful clinical information.

In vivo tests

Skin prick tests

Skin prick tests (SPT) (*Figure 1.1*) have been, and will remain, the gold standard in the diagnosis of allergy. The basic principle of this test is to detect the presence of specific IgE bound to the surface of mast cells and basophils. Upon challenge with the allergen, there is cross-linking between the specific IgE and allergen on

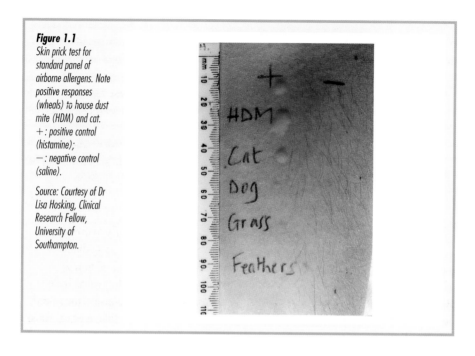

Figure 1.1
Skin prick test for standard panel of airborne allergens. Note positive responses (wheals) to house dust mite (HDM) and cat.
+ : positive control (histamine);
− : negative control (saline).

Source: Courtesy of Dr Lisa Hosking, Clinical Research Fellow, University of Southampton.

the surface of the mast cell/basophil, inducing a process of signal transduction and degranulation. This process results in the release of mast cell products, including histamine, leukotrienes and prostaglandin (PGD_2), which cause the local wheal and flare response.

A drop of the allergen extract and controls (positive (histamine 1–10 mg/ml) and negative (saline or diluent)) are placed on the skin of the volar aspect of the forearm and punctured by means of a 1 mm sterile lancet or a 25 gauge sterile hypodermic needle. The excess solution is absorbed after 30 seconds with an absorbent tissue and the reaction is evaluated after 15–20 minutes. The response is measured as the largest diameter of the wheal and its orthogonal diameter. In the absence of a reaction to the negative control, a reaction of ≥3 × 3 mm is considered as a positive response. It has been shown that a true wheal diameter of 3 mm represents 10 times as much specific IgE as a 2 mm response. If there is a reaction to the diluent due to irritation or dermographism, this value should be subtracted from the responses to the allergens. The results of the SPT should be interpreted carefully, together with the clinical history. Positive tests can be present in an asymptomatic individual and this represents a 'latent allergy' if there is no airway eosinophilia, or termed 'subclinical allergy' when airway eosinophilia is present. It has been shown that, in an asymptomatic individual with a positive reaction to grass pollen, the risk of developing seasonal allergic rhinitis is 10-fold greater than in someone who does not demonstrate a positive reaction. Caution should be exercised, particularly in the interpretation of positive responses to food extracts as only a minority of these patients have a clinical history of food allergy. Most are able to tolerate these foods well without any adverse reactions. In conditions such as oral allergy syndrome, SPT is carried out using the 'prick-prick method' (i.e. the same lancet is used for pricking the fresh fruit/vegetable and then the skin).

Although SPT are a rapid and sensitive means of diagnosing allergy, several studies have shown that reproducibility of the response varies, showing a coefficient of variation of 15% in experienced hands and up to 40% in inexperienced hands, especially when the wheal diameter is <5 mm. Therefore, it has been recommended that these tests are performed in duplicate or quadruplicate.

Intradermal tests are widely used in the USA as an alternative to skin tests and in instances where the clinical history of allergy is strong but the SPT are negative. This involves injecting 0.02–0.05 ml of the extract intradermally to produce a bleb approximately 3 mm in diameter, and a wheal response of >5 mm is considered to be positive. It has been suggested that the response is measured as an erythema rather than a wheal since the former gives a steeper dose-response curve. However, this has not gained widespread acceptance. Although the reproducibility of intradermal testing has been shown to be better than SPT, the former requires greater technical skill. Several factors that affect SPT are summarized in ***Table 1.1***.

Exhaled nitric oxide (NO)

Nitric oxide (NO) is a cytotoxic and cytostatic agent and has been shown to possess immunomodulatory properties. It is a highly reactive molecule with high affinity for iron and iron-sulphur

Table 1.1
Factors affecting SPT.

Factor	Comment
Age	The distribution of skin mast cells is less in the elderly and this can lower the response
Drugs	Antihistamines,* leukotriene receptor antagonists and topical steroids applied to the skin can lower responsiveness. A short course of oral steroids does not affect response
Dermographism	A false positive result

Note:
* With the exception of astemizole (half-life 9.5 days), for other antihistamines it is sufficient to discontinue 4 days prior to SPT. Astemizole must be discontinued for 4 weeks.

containing moieties; consequently it has the capacity to bind to haem, to the enzymes of mitochondrial respiration and DNA synthesis. NO *per se* can exert damaging effects on the cells or could react with superoxide to form peroxynitrite, a powerful oxidant that can then exert cytotoxic effects.

Although the precise role of NO in asthma is not known, recent studies have confirmed that it could be potentially important. The expression of inducible nitric oxide synthase (iNOS), an enzyme important in the generation of NO, has been shown to be significantly upregulated in the bronchial epithelium of nonsteroid-treated asthmatics as opposed to healthy nonatopic controls and steroid-treated asthmatics. Little or only minimal immunoreactivity of iNOS was detectable in the bronchial epithelium of healthy controls. More recently, several groups have validated the measurement of NO in exhaled air using a chemoluminiscent analyser (*Figure 1.2*), and have shown that the level of NO is significantly elevated in nonsteroid-treated asthmatics as opposed to healthy controls and steroid-treated asthmatics (*Figure 1.3*).

Figure 1.2
Measurement of exhaled nitric oxide in the laboratory using a chemiluminiscent analyser.

Source: Courtesy of Mrs C Eames, Research Nurse, University of Southampton.

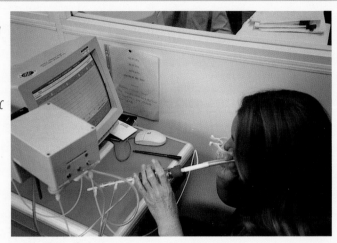

Figure 1.3
Comparison of exhaled NO in asthmatics vs controls. Exhaled NO was significantly elevated in the asthmatic group.

Source: Courtesy of Dr A M Zurek, University of Southampton.

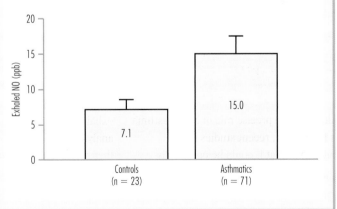

In addition, the levels of exhaled NO are markedly elevated during acute asthma exacerbations and, following treatment with corticosteroids, this drops significantly. Thus exhaled NO has been shown to be a useful surrogate marker in asthma and could be employed for monitoring response to treatment. However, exhaled NO is not specific for asthma since it has been shown to be elevated in patients with adult respiratory distress syndrome, fibrosing alveolitis and pneumonias.

Bronchial reactivity testing

Nonspecific bronchial hyper-responsiveness (BHR) is a characteristic feature of asthma. Several agents (including cold air, carbachol, histamine and methacholine) have been used to study bronchial hyper-responsiveness in asthma. This is mainly a research tool but, nevertheless, is used in certain clinical situations where the clinical diagnosis of asthma is not straightforward. Bronchial reactivity is measured as the dose (cumulative or noncumulative) of bronchoconstrictor, usually histamine or methacholine that induces a 20% fall in FEV_1 (PC_{20} (mg/ml)). During this provocation test, gradually escalating doses of histamine or methacholine are nebulized into the airways and FEV_1 is measured by conventional spirometry at 3 and 5 minutes after each step. The test is terminated when a 20% decline in FEV_1 is achieved, and the bronchoconstriction is reversed by administration of a short-acting β_2 agonist such as salbutamol. PC_{20} is then calculated by interpolation of the last two concentrations that resulted in $\geq$20% drop in FEV_1. *Figure 1.4* illustrates the bronchial hyper-reactivity test graphically in an asthmatic subject. PC_{20} is usually $\leq$8 mg/ml of histamine or methacholine in asthma, and several studies have shown an inverse association between disease severity and PC_{20}, and eosinophil numbers in the airways and PC_{20}, suggesting that PC_{20} could be a reliable marker for disease severity.

Sputum induction

In recent years, sputum induction (*Figure 1.5*) with hypertonic saline has been used extensively as a research tool to investigate airway inflammation in asthma and chronic obstructive pulmonary disease. The main advantage of this procedure is that it is relatively inexpensive, is safe and is less time-consuming than fibreoptic bronchoscopy. Moreover, sputum induction could be performed safely in severe asthmatics in whom bronchoscopy might not be feasible. Recent studies have shown strong

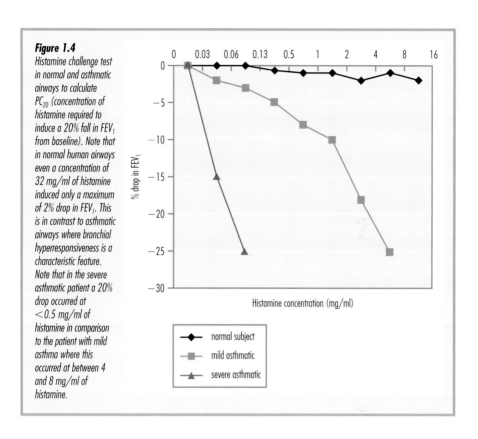

Figure 1.4
Histamine challenge test in normal and asthmatic airways to calculate PC_{20} (concentration of histamine required to induce a 20% fall in FEV_1 from baseline). Note that in normal human airways even a concentration of 32 mg/ml of histamine induced only a maximum of 2% drop in FEV_1. This is in contrast to asthmatic airways where bronchial hyperresponsiveness is a characteristic feature. Note that in the severe asthmatic patient a 20% drop occurred at <0.5 mg/ml of histamine in comparison to the patient with mild asthma where this occurred at between 4 and 8 mg/ml of histamine.

correlations between biomarkers of inflammation measured in the sputum, bronchial wash and bronchoalveolar lavage fluid. Although induced sputum is mainly used for research purposes, it could provide useful information (such as demonstration of lower airway eosinophilia) when the diagnosis of asthma is not straightforward or when monitoring the response to treatment, especially in chronic severe asthmatics on low-dose cyclosporin.

After premedication with salbutamol, a 3%

Figure 1.5
Induced sputum of an asthmatic subject. Note the eosinophilia. Eosinophils show bilobed nucleus with eosinophilic granules in the cytoplasm.

Source: Courtesy of Dr Lisa Hosking, Clinical Research Fellow, University of Southampton.

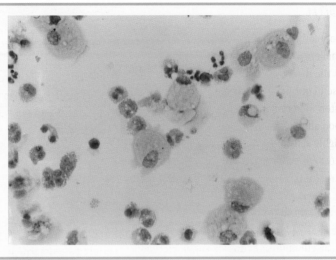

solution of saline is nebulized by means of an ultrasonic nebulizer. Saline is inhaled for 5–30 minutes until an adequate quantity of sputum is expectorated. To prevent salivary contamination and postnasal drip, the patient is advised to rinse his or her mouth and blow his or her nose, respectively. During the inhalation the patient is advised to cough deeply and frequently. The procedure is terminated if FEV_1 falls to greater than 15% of the baseline. Sputum is collected in a plastic petri dish and processed immediately. Equal quantities of 0.1% dithiothreitol are added, followed by equal quantities of Dulbecco's phosphate buffered saline. The sample is shaken gently and placed in a shaking water bath at 37 °C for 15 minutes to ensure complete homogenization. The suspension is then filtered through a gauze (1 mm pore size), the filtrate is centrifuged at 1000 g for 10 minutes and the supernatant is stored at −80 °C for analysis of soluble mediators. The cell pellet is resuspended and the total numbers of non-squamous cells are counted in a modified Neubauer haemocytometer. Cytospin slides are then prepared and stained with Diff-Quick for differential cell counts.

DBPCFC

Double-blind placebo-controlled food challenge (DBPCFC) is the gold standard in the diagnosis of food allergies. It is a useful outpatient procedure that is most often undertaken to refute a history of food allergy, since in studies carried out in highly selected groups of patients only ≤60% of patients have been shown to have positive reactions. The general approach in patients with food allergy is summarized in **Figure 1.6**. There is no need to undertake food challenges if a clear-cut clinical history is supplemented by a positive radioallergosorbent test (RAST) or SPT. However, there are situations in routine practice where multiple foods are implicated in the patient's symptoms and the SPT may show positive reactions to several foods, especially when a panel of allergens is used for skin testing. In such situations, it is best to advise the patient to go on a short but strict elimination diet for 2–4 weeks and to keep a careful record of symptoms during this period. This can be followed by a reintroduction of foods (only when there is no risk of provoking acute life-threatening reactions) one at a time with an interval of at least 2–3 days between each food to see if the symptoms recur and, if they do, whether any temporal relationship exists between

ingestion of the food and onset of symptoms. Some physicians advise a short period of elemental diet if any of the foods in the elimination diet are suspected as being the 'culprit'. If the elimination diet has helped, DPBCFC or open food challenges are performed.

DBPCFC should be performed by an experienced physician with expertise in allergy in a hospital setting, where facilities for immediate resuscitation are readily available. Open food challenges are sometimes carried out merely to reassure certain patients who have strong beliefs that their symptoms are due to food allergy but in whom there is no objective evidence to support the diagnosis.

One of the most challenging and important aspects of DBPCFC is to disguise the food carefully, and this can be done in several ways. Certain foods are available in dehydrated/dried form and these can either be encapsulated in gelatin or mixed in a vehicle such as ice cream, an ice-cold milk shake or any other vehicle that can easily mask the odour and taste. It is often useful to seek the assistance of a dietician. Administration of the food should be undertaken in a graded fashion and the starting quantity should be less than that which is known to provoke symptoms. The dose can then be doubled at intervals

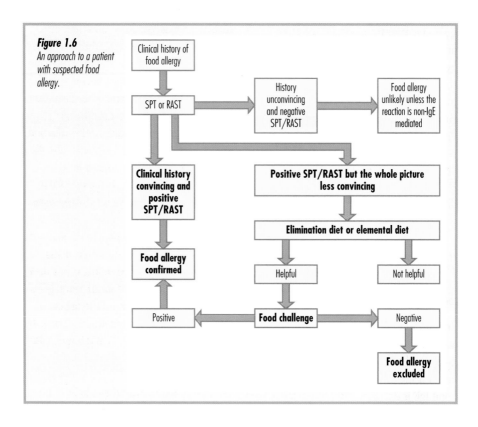

Figure 1.6
An approach to a patient with suspected food allergy.

as dictated by clinical history every 15–60 minutes. The doubling doses should continue until the patient has convincing symptoms, or 8–10 gm dried food or 60–100 gm wet food has been administered as a single dose. If the challenge is negative to this stage, the food must be reintroduced openly in the allergist's office to establish that the patient is able to eat the food without the onset of symptoms.

Certain other important precautions include the avoidance of antihistamines (for the same length of time as for SPT), β_2 agonists, theophylline and cromolyn for

12 hours prior to the challenge. It is optimal to perform the challenges after an overnight fast to eliminate the possibility that previously ingested substances might interfere with the test. It has also been recommended that food and placebo are crossed over several times to ensure the reaction is reproducible. If the symptoms are subjective, it is important to repeat the test after a few months to determine whether or not the problem has persisted.

In vitro tests

Serum total IgE

Immunoglobulin E is secreted by B cells and plasma cells and it is present in all body fluids. It is a useful marker in the investigation of allergic disease. Serum total IgE is extremely low at birth but rises steeply in the first few years of life. It reaches adult levels by the age of 5 years. Since the production of IgE depends on various genetic and environmental factors, the normal distribution curve varies between different countries and, in the UK, the normal range in adults has been estimated to be 1–180 kU/l, with a geometric mean of 21 kU/l. Smokers tend to have higher values than nonsmokers and the majority of atopic individuals have significantly elevated levels although

a small proportion fall within the normal range. Whilst a level of <20 kU/l virtually excludes atopy, a level of >180 kU/l makes the diagnosis more likely. Serum total IgE is also elevated in several other disorders, including parasitic infestations, Wiskott–Aldrich syndrome, HIV infection, alcoholism, hyper-IgE syndrome, allergic bronchopulmonary aspergillosis, Hodgkin's disease, as a result of burns, pemphigoid and rare forms of myelomas.

Serum total IgE is elevated in the majority of patients with allergic asthma, allergic rhinitis and atopic dermatitis. It has been shown that the level of serum total IgE is proportional to the size of the organ affected – it is highest in atopic dermatitis, lowest in allergic rhinitis and intermediate in asthma.

Several immunoassays have been validated for the measurement of total IgE and these include radioimmunoassay (RIA), enzyme-linked immunosorbent assay (ELISA) and the paper radioimmunosorbent test (PRIST). Whilst some tests use solid-phase reagents, others use fluid-phase reagents. These tests are discussed in the following section.

Serum-specific IgE (RAST)

Although a less sensitive method than SPT, *in vitro* measurement of specific IgE in serum may be extremely valuable in certain clinical situations, especially when an SPT cannot be performed. Such situations include dermographism, extensive eczema, the inability of the patient to discontinue antihistamines or when skin testing could carry a risk of provoking serious systemic reactions (rare but reported), as in certain cases of hymenoptera venom and nut allergy.

Serum-specific IgE is measured using a 'sandwich system' (*Figure 1.7*), which involves the addition of the patient's serum to a surface coated with the allergen and the detection of the specific

IgE allergen complex using antihuman-specific IgE. Several assays have been developed based on this principle. In RIA, the anti-IgE is tagged with a radioisotope and the measured radioactivity is proportional to the quantity of specific IgE in the patient's blood. In ELISA (AlaSTAT EIA) the antigen is held in fluid phase and the anti-IgE that is added in the third step of the reaction is labelled with an enzyme. In the final step, a substrate is added to develop a colour reaction, which is detected photometrically as optical density. The concentration of specific IgE is then calculated from the standard curve. In another type of allergosorbent test (CAP-RAST), the allergen is coupled covalently to a cellulose carrier to produce a larger surface area. The patient's serum containing the specific IgE is then added.

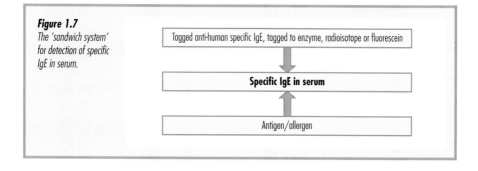

Figure 1.7
The 'sandwich system' for detection of specific IgE in serum.

Tagged anti-human specific IgE, tagged to enzyme, radioisotope or fluorescein

Specific IgE in serum

Antigen/allergen

After the specific IgE binds to the allergen, enzyme-labelled antibodies against IgE are added, and the bound complex is finally incubated with a fluorescent substrate (the developing agent). Fluorescence is then measured in a fluorocounter and the concentration of specific IgE is calculated from the standard curve.

The main disadvantages of *in vitro* systems are that they are less sensitive, time consuming and expensive. Several kits are available commercially for the measurement of specific IgE to aeroallergens, food allergens, insect venom and drugs.

Asthma

2

Introduction

Asthma is one of the commonest disorders encountered in routine clinical practice worldwide both in children and adults. It was once considered a disorder of the airway smooth muscle, causing episodic bronchospasm. However, with the advent of fibreoptic bronchoscopy and developments in molecular biology, it has become easier to gain access into human airways and to study specimens of bronchial mucosa and bronchoalveolavage fluid, and these studies have confirmed that asthma is a chronic inflammatory disorder. The *International Consensus Report for Asthma Management and Prevention*, published in 1993, defined asthma as:

> *a chronic inflammatory disorder of the airways in which many cells play a role, in particular mast cell, eosinophils, and T lymphocytes. In susceptible individuals this inflammation causes recurrent episodes of wheezing, breathlessness, chest tightness and cough particularly at night and/or in the early morning. These symptoms are associated with widespread but variable airflow limitation that is at least partly reversible either spontaneously or with treatment. The inflammation also causes an increase in airway responsiveness to a variety of stimuli.*

The following sections focus on the epidemiology, clinical features and management of asthma. The aetiopathogenesis of asthma is not discussed in this chapter.

Epidemiology

There is now little doubt that the prevalence of atopy and allergic disease has risen worldwide. The International Study of Asthma and Allergies in Childhood (ISAAC) has clearly shown that there was a 20-fold difference in reported asthma symptoms worldwide and that the prevalence of asthma is highest in English-speaking countries, including the UK, Ireland and New Zealand.

Several studies have shown that the prevalence of asthma has risen globally in the last three decades. A study carried out amongst 12-year-old Welsh children has shown an increase in reported asthma from 6 to 12% between 1973 and 1988. In the same study, the prevalence of wheeze was shown to increase from 17 to 22%. A similar survey in Aberdeen school-children in Scotland showed an increase in self-reported asthma from 4.1 to 10.2%. Similarly, prevalence of wheeze and asthma in the past 12 months were 26% and 14%, respectively, amongst

16–50-year-old patients registered in a family practice in Greenwich, UK. This had doubled since a similar study was carried out in Greenwich in 1986. Similar trends have been reported in Europe, North America, Australia and New Zealand.

It has been suggested (and there is mounting evidence for this) that the western 'affluent' life-style is one of the important factors contributing to this rising prevalence. Besides genetic factors, the environment, exposure to indoor allergens (particularly early in life), diet and maternal smoking have been considered to be important determinants in priming the immune system into the development of allergies later on in life. Factors associated with an increased risk of developing asthma are summarized in *Table 2.1*.

In parallel with an overall increase in prevalence rates there is also some evidence to suggest an increase in the severity of the disease. This comes from data on hospital admissions for asthma and on the use of anti-asthma drugs. Studies in the UK, Australia and New Zealand have shown an increase in the use of bronchodilator drugs and inhaled steroids between 1975 and 1981. This could, however, relate to the better or

Table 2.1
Factors contributing to the development of asthma.

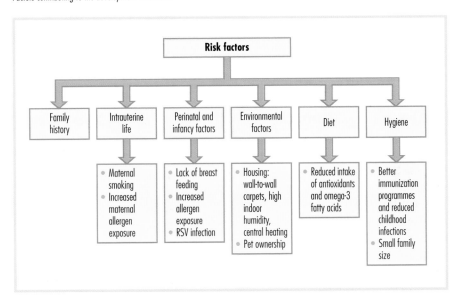

improved care of patients. The increase in severity has been attributed to air pollution, greater house dust mite exposure and occupational factors. Mortality rates from asthma are generally low. In the UK, mortality from asthma showed a steady rise between 1975 (0.59/100 000) and 1987 (0.99/100 000) but then demonstrated a downward trend (0.51/100 000 in 1994). In the UK, a severe thunderstorm in 1994 was associated with the largest outbreak of asthma. Many of the epidemic cases had previously experienced only hay fever, and asthma was probably precipitated in these grass pollen-sensitized individuals by dissemination of small aerosolized particles of grass pollen into the air. In the UK, more deaths from asthma occur during the summer and early autumn than during the winter. This seasonal pattern of asthma deaths has not been observed in

Clinical features

In most cases the diagnosis of asthma is relatively straightforward. Patients usually present with chest tightness, wheeze, shortness of breath and dry cough. Symptoms are usually worse at night and/or early in the morning. Patients sensitive to pollen have seasonal exacerbation of symptoms; those sensitive to animals have episodic symptoms following exposure; and dust mite allergic individuals often have perennial symptoms. The peak expiratory flow rates show characteristic early-morning dips (*Figure 2.1*). This diurnal variation is less apparent after institution of anti-inflammatory therapy. Between 10 and 30% of asthmatics are sensitive to aspirin and nonsteroidal anti-inflammatory drugs (NSAIDs). Other potential trigger factors include exercise, stress, emotion, virus infection, menstruation and sexual intercourse.

A minority of patients present with a dry cough alone, and there is sometimes considerable delay in the diagnosis. In such patients, the important differential diagnoses to consider are postnasal drip due to rhinosinusitis, gastro-oesophageal reflux and lung parenchymal/pleural pathology. Appropriate investigations (including nasal endoscopy, X-rays/CT scans of the sinuses, upper gastrointestinal endoscopy and chest X-ray) will help in the elimination process. In such cases bronchial reactivity tests are often helpful since hyper-reactivity can often be demonstrated in asthma (*Figures 1.4 and 2.2*). Moreover, reversibility in peak flow rate (PEFR) (an increase between 15 and 25%) is demonstrable with a short-acting β_2 agonist in asthmatics.

Management

The three main aspects of asthma management include patient education, the avoidance of allergens and other trigger factors, and pharmacotherapy. There is now little doubt that the institution of this approach reduces asthma morbidity and mortality significantly. In the following sections, each of these aspects is discussed in detail.

Patient education

It is extremely important for patients to have a good insight into their disease,

elderly patients, which probably reflects the importance of seasonal exposure on its severity in younger patients.

Figure 2.1
PEFR in asthma (note the diurnal variation). PEFR shows characteristic early morning dips. This improves after commencement of inhaled corticosteroids.

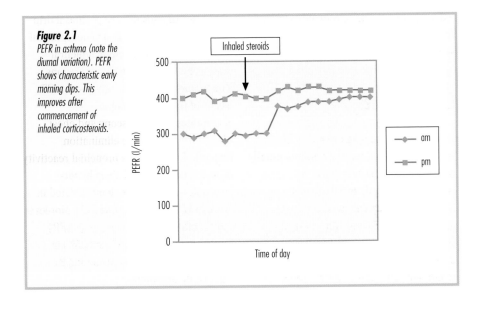

Figure 2.2
Bronchial reactivity in normal subjects and asthmatics. In asthma the PC_{20} to histamine is usually ≤ 8 mg/ml of histamine. This correlates inversely with disease severity, i.e. patients with more severe asthma have a low PC_{20}. In normal subjects PC_{20} is usually >32 mg/ml of histamine.

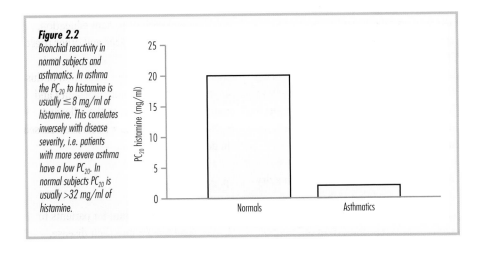

including the benefits of regular pharmacotherapy, allergen avoidance, the adverse effects of air pollution, early aggressive antibiotic therapy for chest infections and a self-management plan for exacerbations (see Appendix I). It is imperative to check inhaler technique and to prescribe the most appropriate inhaler device for patients. Patients with moderate to severe asthma would also benefit from influenza vaccine every winter.

Avoidance of allergens and other triggers

Skin prick tests (SPT) are helpful in identifying the allergens that could trigger and worsen asthma symptoms. Patients with dust mite allergy should institute appropriate measures to reduce the mite load in the indoor environment, including enclosing bedding in impermeable sheets and pillow cases, better indoor ventilation and dehumidification. Patients with pollen allergy should take precautions to avoid exposure during the season by limiting their outdoor activities and they may require escalation of their anti-inflammatory treatment to avoid seasonal exacerbations. Patients with allergy to animals (including cats, dogs or horses) should avoid direct or indirect contact with the respective animal. Allergen is usually present in skin dander, saliva or urine. Some patients may experience

symptoms in response to certain foods, preservatives or drugs (aspirin, NSAIDs and angiotensin-converting enzyme (ACE) inhibitors), and these should be avoided. The adequate treatment of allergic rhinitis has been shown to improve asthma symptoms.

Patients with occupational asthma may have symptoms as a consequence of exposure to certain agents at their workplace. These patients are often symptomatic during the week, and symptoms improve during weekends or periods away from the workplace. Careful clinical history, PEFR monitoring both at work and away from work, and controlled challenges with the occupational agent are necessary to make an accurate diagnosis. Appropriate avoidance measures should be instituted at the workplace to reduce exposure to the noxious agent and, if this is not feasible, patients should be advised about the consequences of continued exposure and about changing their employment. Gastro-oesophageal reflux may provoke asthma symptoms either due to aspiration or laryngeal irritation and this should be treated aggressively with proton pump inhibitors and H_2 blockers. Patients with exercise-induced asthma should be encouraged to exercise normally after taking their bronchodilators. Other potential trigger factors include stress, emotion, menstruation, sexual intercourse and thyrotoxicosis.

Pharmacotherapy

The drugs used in the treatment of asthma are summarized in ***Table 2.2***. A number of national and international guidelines have been developed to help clinicians in the management of asthma. The main approaches underlying these guidelines are to control airway inflammation adequately, to reduce airway remodelling and to prevent irreversible airway narrowing. Most guidelines follow a

Table 2.2
Drugs used in the treatment of asthma.

Bronchodilators (β_2 agonists)
- *Short-acting β_2 agonists:* salbutamol, terbutaline
- *Long-acting β_2 agonists:* salmeterol, eformoterol

Anti-inflammatory drugs
- *Inhaled corticosteroids:* beclomethasone, budesonide, fluticasone
- *Oral corticosteroids:* prednisolone
- *Methylxanthines:* theophylline, aminophylline
- *Antileukotrienes*
- LTRAs: montelukast, zafirlukast
- *5-lipoxygenase inhibitor:* zileuton
- *Cromones:* nedocromil sodium, sodium cromoglycate
- Methotrexate
- Cyclosporin

Novel therapies
- Adenosine receptor ligands
- Anti-CD4 mAb
- Anti-IgE
- *Cytokine monoclonal antibodies (mAb):* IL-4, IL-5, IL-12, IL-13
- *Immunotherapy:* peptide immunotherapy, DNA vaccines, *Mycobacterium vaccae*
- Potassium channel activators
- Selective tryptase inhibitors
- Transcription factor inhibitors
- Type IV phosphodiesterase inhibitors

step-ladder approach to treatment. This should start at a step likely to establish adequate control of the symptoms and, subsequently, treatment should be reduced gradually according to clinical response and PEFR, until a maintenance level is reached. In the following sections, the British Thoracic Society's (BTS) 1997 guidelines (*Table 2.3*) are discussed.

Step 1

This step involves the use of inhaled short-acting β_2 agonists as and when required. If the need for bronchodilator therapy exceeds once a day, regular treatment at a higher step should be instituted. One of the important issues to address is to estimate the patient's threshold for bronchodilator use, especially in those patients with a higher threshold.

Step 2

This involves institution of regular anti-inflammatory therapy with cromones (sodium cromoglycate or nedocromil

---

Table 2.3
Summary of the BTS guidelines for the management of chronic asthma in adults.

Step 1
Inhaled bronchodilators, β_2 agonists ($\leq$1/day)

Step 2
Inhaled bronchodilators as and when required + anti-inflammatory therapy (cromones or beclomethasone or budesonide 400 ug/d) (? LTRAs* instead of inhaled steroids)

Step 3
Step 2 plus increase dose of inhaled steroids, or add long-acting β_2 agonists, or LTRAs

Step 4
High-dose inhaled steroids + long-acting β_2 agonists + LTRAs or theophylline or anticholinergic

Step 5
Step 4 + oral steroids ± immunosuppressive agents (cyclosporin/methotrexate)

* Currently in the UK, LTRAs are licensed only for treatment of asthma not adequately controlled by inhaled steroids or in EIA or aspirin-induced asthma.

sodium) or inhaled corticosteroids (100–400 µg twice daily). Beclomethasone is equivalent to budesonide at the same dose but to fluticasone at half the dose when given by metered dose inhaler (MDI). There is now considerable debate regarding the introduction of leukotriene receptor antagonists (LTRAs) such as montelukast or zafirlukast at this stage, but these were not included in the 1997 BTS guidelines. These drugs have, however, received approval to be introduced at step 2 in the USA and it is conceivable that this issue will be addressed in the near future in the UK after the results of the long-term efficacy of LTRAs become available from ongoing clinical studies.

Step 3

This step involves escalating the dose of inhaled corticosteroids or the introduction of long-acting β_2 agonists, such as salmeterol or eformoterol. Recent studies have shown better control of asthma symptoms with the introduction of a long-acting β_2 agonist rather than increasing the dose of inhaled steroids. However, increasing the dose of inhaled steroids seemed to reduce asthma exacerbations significantly. Hence, strategies at this stage should be tailored to the individual patients, depending upon their clinical history.

Step 4

This involves a combination of a higher dose of inhaled steroids together with a long-acting β_2 agonist. Other drugs to be considered at this stage include theophylline or anticholinergic drugs, such as ipratopium bromide. Theophylline is more widely used in the USA and the rest of the world than in the UK. The main concern with this drug is its narrow therapeutic index and its potential drug interactions (**Figure 2.3**). When used carefully, however, it is extremely effective owing to its bronchodilator and anti-inflammatory properties. It is particularly useful in alleviating nocturnal symptoms.

LTRAs have been licensed in the UK to be prescribed for patients with moderate asthma whose symptoms are inadequately controlled with inhaled steroids. Their role should be evaluated carefully at steps 2–4 of the current guidelines.

Step 5

This step involves the introduction of regular oral steroids. Patients are often commenced on a higher dose that is likely to control their symptoms, and the dosage is gradually titrated to a maintenance level after careful evaluation of clinical response and PEFR charts. Before the institution of oral steroids it is

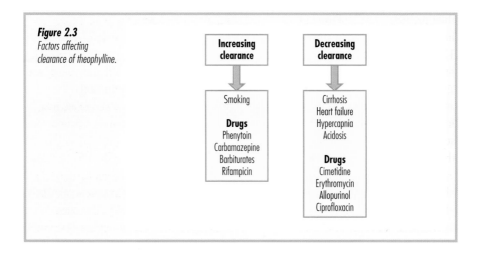

Figure 2.3
Factors affecting
clearance of theophylline.

Increasing clearance	Decreasing clearance
Smoking	Cirrhosis
	Heart failure
Drugs	Hypercapnia
Phenytoin	Acidosis
Carbamazepine	
Barbiturates	**Drugs**
Rifampicin	Cimetidine
	Erythromycin
	Allopurinol
	Ciprofloxacin

extremely important to re-evaluate the patient's compliance, any unidentified trigger factors and psychosocial issues. If long-term therapy seems essential, patients should be advised about the risks (the development of osteoporosis, in particular). Appropriate preventative measures include regular exercise, calcium/vitamin D supplements, biphosphonates and hormone replacement therapy in postmenopausal patients. If the patients require extremely high doses of oral steroids, alternative measures include immunosuppressive therapy, such as cyclosporin or methotrexate. Such patients should be referred to clinicians who have experience of the management of chronic severe asthma.

Novel asthma therapies currently under evaluation are listed in *Table 2.2*.

Management of chronic severe asthma

In a small proportion of patients, asthma may be difficult to control even with the regime at step 5 of the BTS guidelines. A systematic clinical approach would be of utmost importance in such patients, and it is important to check treatment compliance, inhaler technique, environmental triggers, psychosocial issues and concomitant conditions (including gastro-oesophageal reflux and sinusitis). Patients who demonstrate reversibility with salbutamol, who have prebronchodilator morning FEV_1 <70% of their predicted rate and who fail to increase this prebronchodilator FEV_1 by 15% after at least a one week course of prednisolone 40 mg/d are defined as 'glucocorticosteroid-resistant (GR) asthmatics'. Pharmacokinetic studies are indicated if a patient fails to respond to steroids or is unable to tolerate doses less than 20 mg on alternate days. This evaluation can identify abnormal pharmacokinetics, such as rapid elimination (most frequent), drug interactions (concominant use of anticonvulsants, such as phenytoin sodium, carbamazepine or phenobarbitone) or poor absorption.

Molecular studies have revealed two types of GR asthmatics:

Type I   Reduced glucocorticoid receptor (GCR) binding. These patients have severe side-effects from long-term steroid therapy.

Type II   Reduced GCR numbers. These patients do not experience any long-term side-effects of steroid therapy.

There are several anecdotal reports regarding the efficacy of several anti-inflammatory agents, such as cyclosporin, methotrexate, gold and intravenous gammaglobulin, in patients who have difficulty in controlling asthma and who have steroid-resistant asthma. Further case-control studies are required in larger patient populations to identify clearly the usefulness of these agents in the management of chronic severe asthma.

Management of asthma in pregnancy

At least one third of women with asthma experience worsening of their symptoms during pregnancy. Poorly controlled asthma could result in increased perinatal mortality, prematurity and low birth weight due to hypoxia of the foetus. Short-acting β_2 agonists, inhaled corticosteroids, theophylline and sodium cromoglycate are not associated with foetal abnormalities. If systemic steroids are indicated prior to delivery, prednisolone/methyl prednisolone are preferable to hydrocortisone/dexamethasone since the former do not significantly cross the placenta. The safety of LTRAs in pregnancy is not yet established and these agents should not be used. Acute attacks must be treated aggressively with adequate oxygenation, nebulized β_2 agonists and systemic corticosteroids when necessary.

Modalities of aerosol drug delivery in asthma

The introduction of pressurized metered dose inhalers (MDIs) (pMDIs) in 1956 revolutionalized the management of asthma. Since then considerable advances have taken place in aerosol science leading to the development of a number of inhaler devices. This has caused a great deal of confusion amongst clinicians and patients and it is important to understand the pros and cons of individual inhaler devices and to determine which is the most suitable for the patient. The classification of currently available delivery systems is summarized in *Table 2.4*.

A detailed description of these devices is beyond the scope of this book but some salient feature are discussed below.

pMDIs

Most pMDIs contain the active drug together with propellants and surfactants that enable aerosolization of the drug. With good inhaler technique drug deposition in the lungs varies between 10 and 15%. Considerable skill and co-ordination are required to ensure good drug deposition. This can be difficult in children, elderly people or patients with arthritis because it involves the small joints of the fingers. In addition, initial paradoxical bronchoconstriction can occur even with bronchodilators. The problem of co-ordination can be overcome

Table 2.4
Inhaler devices in asthma.

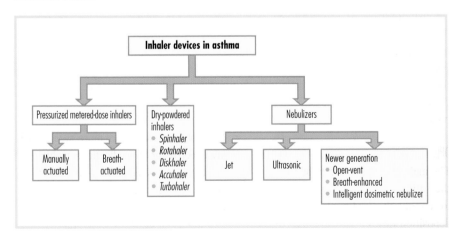

by the use of a 'breath-actuated device' which is triggered by the patient's inspiration at a low flow rate.

Under the terms of the Montreal Protocol, the use of chlorofluorocarbons (CFCs) as propellants is gradually being phased out in all MDIs with hydrofluoroalkanes (HFAs). Drug deposition with HFAs differs from chlorofluoroalkanes (CFAs). For example, a better lung deposition from some CFC-free inhalers (such as the beclomethasone product Qvar) allows the prescribed dose to be halved.

pMDI with spacer

The problem of co-ordination with pMDIs can also be overcome by introducing a large volume spacer with a one-way valve mechanism. With this system the patient can actuate the MDI and breathe tidally through the spacer. This will ensure better deposition in the lungs and will prevent oropharyngeal impaction, thus reducing both local and systemic adverse effects in the case of inhaled steroids. The main disadvantage of this system is the bulkiness of the apparatus.

DPIs

The main principle underlying DPIs is that they utilize the patient's inspiratory force to generate the drug aerosol. Drug lung deposition varies between 10 and 30%.

Various DPIs are currently available, including the spinhaler, rotahaler, turbuhaler, diskhaler and the diskus device. Both the spinhaler and rotahaler require individual loading of the capsule into the device before each inhalation. The turbuhaler and diskus (accuhaler) are multidose inhalers containing several doses preloaded in a reservoir. As with pMDIs, oropharyngeal impaction and cough can be a problem in some patients. To reduce systemic absorption and oral thrush formation, all patients taking inhaled steroids *via* an MDI or DPI should be advised to gargle after each inhalation.

Nebulizers

Nebulizers enable the rapid delivery of a greater dosage of the drug into the lungs as may perhaps be required during an acute asthma attack. They vary greatly in the droplet size they generate, their nebulization time and drug output. Different drugs nebulized from the same nebulizer will not have identical output characteristics.

Jet nebulizers, which are more widely used, are effective for all medications, including particulate suspensions as in the case of corticosteroids. Ultrasonic nebulizers use a piezoelectric crystal to produce high-frequency sound waves, which then generate aerosol dispersion. They are not as effective as jet nebulizers and cannot be used to deliver corticosteroids.

Appendix I: A written self-management plan for an adult patient with mild-moderate asthma

The usual PEFR is 450–500 lit/min. Usual medication: Ventolin MDI 2 puffs p.r.n. + Becotide 100 MDI 2 puffs b.d.

*PEFR <350:** Ventolin 2 puffs q.d.s. + Becotide 100 2 puffs q.d.s. and monitor PEFR and symptoms carefully.

*PEFR <250:** Commence tablets. Prednisolone 40 mg/d and monitor PEFR and symptoms carefully. Once PEFR returns to normal, tail down prednisolone by 5 mg/d every 3 days.

PEFR <200: Go to emergency department.

* In case of any respiratory tract infections, patients are advised to start antibiotics early.

Further reading

Barnes PJ, Rodger IW, Thompson NC, eds. *Asthma* (3rd edn) (Academic Press, 1998).

The BTS guidelines on the management of asthma. *Thorax* 1997; **52 (suppl 4)**.

Clark T, Rees J, eds. *Practical Management of Asthma* (3rd edn) (Martin Dunitz, London, 1998).

Cockrane GM, Jackson WF, Rees JP. *Asthma: Current Perspectives* (Mosby-Wolfe, London, 1996).

Global Initiative for Asthma. National Heart, Lung and Blood Institute Publication 95-3659 (National Institute of Health, London, January 1995).

Lordan JL, Holgate ST. Recent developments in the pathogenesis of asthma. *J R Coll Physicians Lond* 1999; **33:** 418–24.

Phillips K, Harrison TW, Tattersfield A. New asthma drugs. *J R Coll Physicians Lond* 1999; **33:** 425–30.

Rhinitis

3

Introduction

Rhinitis is one of the most frequent conditions for which patients consult their family physician. Rhinitis is an inflammatory response of the nasal mucosa to various stimuli, both allergic and nonallergic. It is characterized by symptoms of nasal congestion, sneezing, nasal pruritus, rhinorrhoea and hyposmia. Allergic rhinitis typically affects 20% of the population and is associated with a history consistent with immediate hypersensitivity and a family history of atopy. In a study examining an adult population in London, 16% of patients seen had allergic rhinitis, of which 8% had perennial symptoms and 6% had both perennial and seasonal complaints.

A child has a 70% risk of developing allergic rhinitis if both parents have a family history of atopy. The risk is reduced to 50% if only one parent has atopy. The onset of allergic rhinitis appears to be higher in the primary school age-group and peaks during the second decade of life. Symptoms of allergic rhinitis are common and persist in the first four decades of life, but usually improve after the age of 50 years. It is seen infrequently in older people. Individuals with mild and seasonal symptoms are most likely to have remissions, but only 5–10% of patients tend to overcome their problems within 5 years.

Differential diagnosis

It is difficult to differentiate between allergic and nonallergic rhinitis, especially when viral infections occur during the peak of an allergy season. Many elderly patients are convinced they have allergies because of pseudo-allergic responses (such as vasomotor rhinitis). Allergic conditions are divided into seasonal (seasonal allergic rhinitis or SAR) and perennial (perennial allergic rhinitis or PAR), but it is also worth considering occupational rhinitis as a subdivision of perennial rhinitis (*Table 3.1*).

The differentiation between seasonal and perennial conditions is not always straightforward. For example, if an individual with SAR is susceptible to a variety of pollens that are produced at different times of the year, symptoms can persist for many months, giving the appearance of a perennial condition.

Occupational allergic rhinitis occurs as a response to aeroallergens in the workplace and they can affect patients all year round. Common causes are laboratory animals, grain, wood dusts (particularly hardwoods), chemicals and solvents.

The key points in the clinical history of a patient that would be helpful in the diagnosis of rhinitis are as follows:

1 *Symptoms*
   - Onset: seasonality, duration, time of the day.
   - Character: type of discharge, itchiness, runny nose, sneezing, congestion.
   - Symptoms from other systems (asthma, urticaria).
2 *Triggers*
   - Environment: home/work; indoor/outdoor association; heating, damp, mould, furniture, smoking, pets, plants, ventilation.
   - Trips, holidays, day care for children.
   - Sports, hobbies.
   - Foods.
3 *Feeding history* (for children).
4 *Past medical history* Atopy, trauma, response to treatment.
5 *Family history* History of allergic diseases.

Table 3.1
The differential diagnosis of rhinitis.

Allergic	Infectious	Noninfectious, nonallergic	
Seasonal	*Acute*	*Systemic*	*Mechanical factors*
Perennial	• Viral	• Primary defect in mucus	• Deviated septum
Occupational	• Bacterial	– Cystic fibrosis	• Hypertrophic turbinates
	• Fungal	– Young's syndrome	• Adenoidal hypertrophy
		– Primary ciliary dyskinesia	• Foreign body
	Chronic	• Immunological	• Choanal atresia
	• Viral	– SLE	
	• Bacterial	– Rheumatoid arthritis	*Other causes*
	• Fungal	• Endocrine/hormonal	• Polyps
	• Protozoal	– Hypothyroidism	• Idiopathic
	• Parasitic	– Pregnancy	• Cholinergic (vasomotor)
		– Old man's drip	• Nonallergic rhinitis with
		• Granulomatous disease	eosinophilia (NARES)
		– Wegener's granulomatosis	• Occupational
		– Sarcoidosis	• Drug-induced
		– Rhinoscleromatosis	(medicamentosa)
		– Midline granuloma	• Irritants
		– Amyloidosis	• Food
		• Diabetes mellitus	• Emotional
		• Antibody deficiency	• Atrophic
		• AIDS	
		• Tumours	

The symptoms and history that can differentiate allergic from nonallergic causes are summarized in *Table 3.2*.

The typical allergic symptoms include sneezing, runny nose (rhinorrhoea), itchy nose, eyes or throat (palatal itch) and nasal congestion, which may be present all or in part. The associated symptoms of chronic mouth breathing, postnasal discharge, hyposmia and cough may also be present. The patient may develop complications with symptoms of recurrent rhinosinusitis or recurrent secretory otitis media secondary to chronic nasal obstruction and eustachian tube dysfunction.

Seasonal allergic rhinitis is the most readily recognized form. The symptoms of most tree sensitivities are present in the early spring, and grass sensitivity is present when the grasses pollinate in the late spring or early summer (*Figure 3.1*). Hay fever is usually accompanied by the production of ragweed pollen in late summer (*Figure 3.1*). In contrast, perennial allergies are all year round and are caused mostly by indoor allergens. Perennial rhinitis could be secondary to exposure to indoor pets, house dust and house dust mites, animal feathers, moulds and cockroaches.

Table 3.2
Differentiation of allergic from nonallergic rhinitis.

	Allergic rhinitis	Nonallergic rhinitis
Onset of symptoms	Early in life	Usually after the age of 30
Family history	At least one parent affected	Negative
Seasonality	Common	Uncommon
Triggers	Suspected allergens identifiable	Symptoms precipitated by irritants/weather changes
Symptoms	Nasal, ocular, throat pruritus No fever or myalgias	Other systems not affected 'Flu-like' symptoms (infectious origin)
On examination	Nasal turbinates moist, slightly blue	Erythematous, inflamed, often dry mucosa

Figure 3.1
Pollen calendar for the UK.

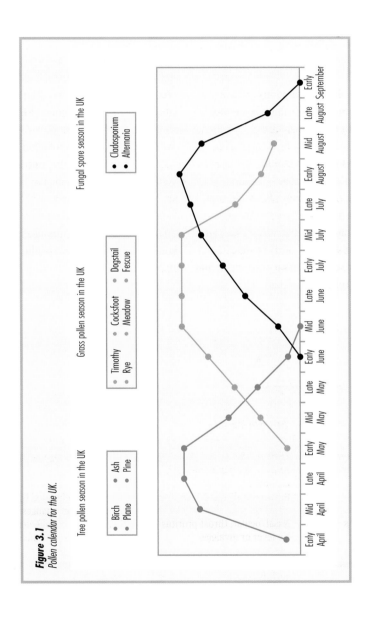

It is important to inquire about the association of acute symptoms with exposure to specific allergens during specific activities, such as to house dust mites when vacuuming, to animals, to mould spores when harvesting or to leaves or grass pollen when gardening. Frequently, unsuspected occupational allergens can stimulate an IgE-mediated response and inquiries should be made about the working environment. Examples of occupational aeroallergens include commercial flours used in baking and food preparation and aerosolized latex rubber allergen which can be a source of respiratory symptoms in hospital personnel who have significant exposure to latex in such areas as operating rooms. Furthermore, sports or leisure activities may be exacerbating factors for rhinitis. Food allergies rarely cause allergic rhinitis in adults. *Table 3.3* summarizes some relevant points in clinical history in the evaluation of patients with allergic rhinitis.

Physical examination

The patient with acute allergic rhinitis may appear quite uncomfortable and distressed and may be mouth breathing. Children with chronic allergic rhinitis

Table 3.3
Points to consider in the evaluation of patients with allergic rhinitis.

- Is there a family history of atopy, such as allergic rhinitis, asthma or eczema?
- Is there a personal history of atopy, such as eczema during infancy and childhood?
- Can the patient provide a detailed chronology and description of the symptoms?
- Information about the home environment (heating, bedding materials, carpets, damp, mould, the condition of the air, pets)
- Are there increasing symptoms during a particular season, during activity such as vacuuming, gardening or in the presence of irritants and pollutants, such as tobacco smoke, potpourri, household chemicals?
- What are the hobbies, sports and leisure activities and are they related to the aggravation of symptoms?
- Are the nasal symptoms isolated or are there concomitant signs from other parts of the upper airways, such as sinuses or ears? Is there a history of lower airway, ocular or dermatological disease, such as bronchial asthma, conjunctivitis, eczema or urticaria?

may exhibit facial pallor as well as dental malocclusion with a high-arched palate. Rhinorrhoea is typically clear, although, rarely, the density of eosinophils and neutrophils imparts a yellowish-green colour to the secretions. Other common findings include the following:

- *Allergic salute*, which is common in children, involves using the palm of the hand in an upward thrust of the nares, thereby relieving itching and opening the nasal airway. This can lead to the development of the 'allergic crease', a hyperpigmented or hypopigmented groove at the junction of the tip of the nose and the more rigid nasal bridge.
- *Allergic gape* or continuous open-mouth breathing, usually a result of nasal blockage.
- *Dennie–Morgan folds*, a wrinkle just beneath the lower eyelids that is present from early infancy and is associated with atopic dermatitis and allergic rhinitis.
- *Allergic shiners* or dark discoloration in the orbital-palpebral grooves beneath the lower eyelids. These are probably secondary to venous stasis caused by mucosal oedema of the nose and sinuses.
- *Cobblestoning* (or bands of lymphoid hyperplasia on the posterior pharynx)

is usually a result of chronic postnasal drainage.

- *Common complications*, such as otitis media, sinusitis or nasal polyps, should be sought as part of the routine examination.
- In examining the *mouth*, malocclusion or a high-arched palate associated with chronic mouth breathing, tonsillar hypertrophy, lymphoid 'streaking' in the oropharynx, pharyngeal postnasal discharge and dysosmia might be present.
- In addition to nasal symptoms, *eye symptoms*, such as tearing, oedema, scleral or conjunctival injection, may be present, especially in patients with pollen and animal allergies. A flare-up of pre-existing *eczema* can occur and occasionally contact urticaria might be present. Also signs of *asthma* should be looked for.

The nasal mucosa in all patients with rhinitis may be examined by insertion of an otoscope (with a nasal speculum tip of appropriate size attached), first into one nostril and then into the other. The speculum should be inserted gently because the septum may be quite tender. Elevating the end of the nose with the other hand provides a better view of the nasal passage. A nasal speculum with a headlight or a flexible fibreoptic endoscope will allow an even more detailed examination of the nose.

Nasal examination of the patient with allergic rhinitis may be normal or may reveal watery mucus on the epithelial surface. The mucosa can be inflamed, with a bluish-grey appearance when the mucosal oedema is severe. Occasionally, the mucosa can be hyperaemic. Inferior turbinates may appear polypoid due to oedema and may be confused with nasal polyps, which have a characteristic greyish 'peeled grape' appearance. Nasal polyps can easily be distinguished from nasal turbinates as they appear glistening and opaque and are insensitive to touch (unlike the turbinate). Polyps may be differentiated from severely oedematous mucosa by applying a small amount of a topical vasoconstrictor, such as phenylephrine, to the mucosa and re-examining 5–10 minutes later. Nasal polyps will not shrink in size after topical vasoconstrictor has been applied, unlike oedematous mucosa. Also, nasal polyps tend to be mobile and insensitive to touch, whereas an oedematous mucosa is extremely sensitive to touch (or manipulation) and is not mobile. The nasal septum should be inspected carefully for any significant deviation as well as for any pre-existing lesions, such as perforation. Useful investigations in the diagnosis of allergic rhinitis are summarized in **Table 3.4**.

The use of laboratory evaluation to determine a cause should be limited. Skin testing and radioallergosorbent (RAST) testing should be used in conjunction with personal history and clinical examination to identify the possible aetiological-allergic factor. Skin tests are positive in 10–15% of asymptomatic individuals. Over-reliance on mildly positive RAST tests for diagnosis and therapy may erroneously perpetuate the impression of an allergy to a specific factor. Such a false impression is difficult to change in patients who are seeking a cause for their long-lasting complaints. Provocation-neutralization testing, set end-point titration and RAST for specific IgE for food antigens or *Candida* are all controversial and have not been shown to provide reliable evidence of allergy.

Acute or chronic sinusitis is frequently associated with acute or chronic infectious rhinitis. The assessment of infectious rhinitis requires investigation and treatment of coexisting sinusitis.

Table 3.4
Investigations in the diagnosis of allergic rhinitis.

Diagnostic tests in allergic rhinitis	Objective methods of measuring nasal patency
Skin tests	Nasal airway resistance
In vitro tests (e.g. RAST)	Passive anterior rhinomanometry
Total IgE	Active anterior rhinomanometry
Blood eosinophilia	Active posterior rhinomanometry
Nasal cytology	Postnasal rhinomanometry
Rhinomanometry	Plethysmography method
Rhinoscopy – flexible and rigid	Oscillometry method
Imaging – radiology and CT	Acoustic reflection rhinomanometry
Tests of mucociliary clearance	Rhinostereometry
Nasal provocation challenge	Nasal peak flow

Nonallergic rhinitis with eosinophilia syndrome (NARES)

The nonallergic rhinitis with eosinophilia syndrome (NARES) is characterized by perennial or seasonal nasal congestion, sneezing or watery rhinorrhoea with intermittent itching of the ears, palate and nose. Triggers may include irritants, such as perfume or smoke, and changes in the weather. Physical examination reveals a nasal mucosa that is pale and polypoid changes may be observed. Profuse secretions containing large numbers of eosinophils may be present during symptomatic periods. These patients have

negative skin tests for aeroallergens and negative RAST. In a study evaluating patients with negative skin testing, 33% of patients had NARES (based on a nasal smear revealing >5% nasal eosinophils), and 61% had vasomotor rhinitis.

Cholinergic/vasomotor rhinitis

Vasomotor rhinitis consists of a combination of symptoms, including sneezing and watery rhinorrhoea with or without nasal congestion that develop rapidly but also resolve quickly. Typically, onset of symptoms can be related to rapid changes in outside temperature. Although it is described in the literature as a syndrome with watery rhinorrhoea and sneezing but without nasal congestion, in everyday practice it is common to see patients with a combination of the above plus nasal congestion that cannot be attributed to infection or allergy and who do not fit into any other of the categories of rhinitis rather than vasomotor. It is useful to categorize these patients for clinical purposes as having nonallergic vasomotor rhinitis, although this classification continues to be far from satisfactory in defining the aetiology of their symptoms.

Drug-induced rhinitis (rhinitis medicamentosa)

Several medications are associated with nasal symptoms. Aspirin and nonsteroidal anti-inflammatory drugs (NSAIDs) promote rhinitis associated with asthma but these are not IgE-mediated. Beta-blockers, terazosin, reserpine, methyldopa and oral contraceptives can produce nasal congestion. Perhaps the best known side-effect is rebound nasal congestion that occurs with abuse of topical nasal decongestants (rhinitis medicamentosa). Patients with rhinitis medicamentosa have a history of chronic nasal congestion, especially at night, characterized by short periods of relief following the use of a nasal

decongestant spray. These patients often have an associated underlying rhinitis that, in the first place, leads them to the use of the decongestant spray. It is not known when patients develop rebound congestion, but typically they notice they have to use the topical decongestant more frequently because of shorter duration of relief.

Physical examination of the nasal passages usually reveals a 'beefy' red mucosa with minimal secretions. Treatment consists of weaning the patient off the nasal decongestant spray. The differential diagnosis should include cocaine abuse, especially in patients who present with rhinitis associated with nasal septal perforation.

Pharmacotherapy

Antihistamines

Antihistamines have been used in the treatment of allergic rhinitis for more than 50 years. Their therapeutic effect is based on the blockade of H_1 histamine receptors located on the nasal vasculature and nerve endings. They act by blocking the activity of histamine without initiating a response, an action that is both competitive and reversible. H_1-receptor antagonists effectively inhibit histamine-induced vasodilatation, increased capillary permeability, smooth muscle constriction and increased glandular secretions and treat rhinitis by reducing sneezing and rhinorrhoea. However, they have little or no effect on nasal congestion. Because antihistamines can effectively block receptor sites before histamine release, the best results are obtained when they are administered on a regular basis and as a prophylactic measure to allergic persons prior to allergen exposure. More recently, *in vitro* studies have identified certain anti-inflammatory effects of second-generation antihistamines, including a decrease in the expression of intercellular adhesion molecule (ICAM)-1 and eosinophil chemotaxis.

Second-generation H_1-receptor antagonists can be distinguished from first-generation drugs by their greater affinity for H_1 receptors, with a slower dissociation rate and a longer duration of action. They also lack appreciable central nervous system (CNS) and anticholinergic effects compared with their first-generation counterparts.

All the first-generation and most of the second-generation antihistamines are metabolized by the hepatic cytochrome P-450 system. Half-life values range from less than 24 hours for terfenadine, loratadine and cetirizine, to 9.5 days for astemizole and its active metabolites. It can be even further prolonged in elderly patients, in patients with hepatic dysfunction and in patients receiving other P-450 inhibitors, such as ketoconazole or erythromycin. All antihistamines are readily absorbed and reach peak concentrations 2 hours after oral administration. However, the high tissue penetrance of the drug and its active metabolites prolong its effectiveness even after the serum concentrations have declined.

A list of products is given in *Table 3.5* and their adverse effects in *Table 3.6*.

Cautions and contraindications

Antihistamines should be used with caution in prostatic hypertrophy, glaucoma, epilepsy and hepatic impairment. Astemizole, mizolastine and terfenadine should be avoided in significant liver dysfunction. Many antihistamines should be avoided in porphyria, although chlorpheniramine and cetirizine are thought to be safe.

Oral and nasal decongestants

Ephedrine nasal drops are the safest sympathomimetic drug and are very

Table 3.5
Formulation and dosage of H_1-receptor antagonists.

Drug name	Formulation	Dose	Paediatric use
Acrivastine	Semprex caps 8 mg	8 mg t.d.s.	≥12 years
Astemizole	Hismanal tabs 10 mg	10 mg o.d.	≥12 years
	Hismanal susp. 5 mg/5 ml	5 mg o.d.	6–12 years
Cetirizine	Zirtek tabs 10 mg	10 mg o.d.	≥6 years
	Zirtek oral solution 5 mg/5 ml	5 mg o.d. or 2.5 mg b.d.	2–6 years
Fexofenadine	Telfast tabs 120 mg	120 mg o.d.	≥12 years
Loratadine	Clarityn tabs 10 mg	10 mg o.d.	≥30 kg
	Clarityn syr 5 mg/5 ml	5 mg o.d.	2–12 years, ≥30 kg
Mizolastine	Mizollen tabs 10 mg	10 mg o.d.	≥12 years

Table 3.6
Side-effects of first-generation antihistamines.

Drowsiness
Psychomotor impairment
Headache
Anticholinergic effects:

- Dry mouth
- Impotence
- Urinary retention
- Gastrointestinal disturbances

Impairment of ability to perform tasks
Cardiovascular effects:

- Arrhythmia
- Hypotension
- Sudden death

Hypersensitivity reactions

effective for several hours. Xylometazoline, oxymetazoline and phenylephrine are more potent with longer activity but are most likely to cause rebound syndrome. A vasoconstrictor spray should be used very cautiously and for a limited amount of time (5–7 days) because of the onset of rhinitis medicamentosa. Its use should be limited in specific conditions, such as sinusitis, before the use of topical steroids, in order to ensure their optimal distribution in the nose, and before professional or other activities.

It is vital to educate patients about the correct usage of topical vasoconstrictors as their abuse could lead to severe intoxication. Long-term treatment with an intranasal α-adrenoreceptor agonist can cause rhinitis medicamentosa characterized by nasal congestion, increased nasal irritability and a dry and burning nose. When this occurs the medication should be gradually reduced over 7–10 days with the concomitant use of intranasal steroids to reduce the inflammation. They can also cause tachyphylaxis when they are used frequently in progressively shorter intervals.

Adrenergic agonists (such as pseudoephedrine and phenylephrine) can be administered orally with significant improvement in allergic and nonallergic rhinitis. The lowest dose needed should be used to relieve nasal congestion.

A-adrenergic agonists can also be used in combination with antihistamines in allergic rhinitis. The effects of these drugs supplement each other to the symptomatic relief of rhinitis, and their side-effects on the CNS are neutralized. Nasal decongestants are listed in *Table 3.7*.

Ipratropium bromide

Intranasal ipratropium bromide has been used for both allergic and nonallergic rhinitis and is helpful in treating both rhinorrhoea and postnasal discharge. It also has been shown to be safe and effective for children over 6 years of age in treating perennial nonallergic rhinitis. Ipratropium bromide does not produce rebound symptoms and no significant adverse effects have been reported. However, ipratropium bromide has no effect on relieving nasal congestion or in modifying the allergic reaction.

Cromolyn sodium and nedocromil sodium

Cromones are mast-cell stabilizers that can be used regularly (four times a day) as a pretreatment. They give dose-related protection against both the immediate and the late response of an allergic reaction and are generally well tolerated by patients, especially with mild nasal irritation or burning. They may be used prophylactically for unavoidable challenge exposures, for example, when a

Table 3.7
Decongestants for rhinitis.

	Drug name	Formulation	Dose	Paediatric use
Topical	Pseudoephedrine	Sudafed/Galpseud tabs 60 mg	60 mg up to 4 times daily	≥12 years
	Hydrochloride	Sudafed elixir 30 mg/5 ml	10 ml up to 4 times daily	≥12 years
Systemic	Ephedrine	Ephedrine nasal drops	1–2 drops, 3–4 times daily	≥3 months
	Xylometazoline	Xylometazoline nasal drops	2–3 drops 2–3 times daily	≥12 years
		Xylometazoline nasal drops paediatric	1–2 drops, 1–2 times daily (max. 7 days)	≥3 months

cat-sensitive patient is obliged to visit a home where there is a cat or for a few weeks before the pollen season. For effective topical nasal use, the medication has to be used at least four times a day. One advantage of the use of topical nasal cromolyn is that no significant adverse reactions have been reported. Local side-effects occur in fewer than 10% of patients and most commonly involve sneezing, nasal stinging, burning or irritation.

Of the new mast-cell stabilizing agents, nedocromil sodium has also been shown to decrease mast cell numbers, rhinorrhoea, nasal congestion and sneezing. Furthermore, it has been shown to have additional pharmacological characteristics, including inhibition of eosinophil influx.

Intranasal corticosteroids

Topical corticosteroids are considered the gold standard of therapy for the symptoms of allergic rhinitis. They are effective in reducing nasal blockage, itching, sneezing and rhinorrhoea in allergic and nonallergic noninfectious rhinitis. They are most effective when commenced several days before allergen or irritant exposure and should therefore be used on a regular rather than an 'as-needed' basis. The local application of intranasal steroids virtually eliminates any systemic side-effects. Local side-effects, although uncommon, include nasal irritation and bleeding, which are often due to the drug delivery device or to the local effect of the spray rather than being a side-effect of the drug *per se*. Formulations of currently available intranasal corticosteroids are listed in ***Table 3.8***.

Antileukotrienes

The role of cysteinyl leukotrienes in the pathophysiology of asthma and allergic rhinitis is well established. Studies with leukotriene antagonists, such as pranlukast, montelukast and zafirlukast, have shown promising results in their ability to alleviate the symptoms of allergic rhinitis. These studies demonstrate rapid onset of symptomatic relief that is similar to that of antihistamines, whilst the combination of leukotriene antagonists with antihistamines provided superior symptom control than either drug alone in allergic rhinitis. However, short-term and long-term studies are required to establish the role of these novel agents in the

management of allergic rhinitis, particularly a comparison of their effects with intranasal corticosteroids. Because a significant proportion of patients with asthma also have allergic rhinitis and because the treatment of rhinitis improves asthma symptoms, it might be logical to use these agents as an adjunct to topical nasal steroids to control both upper and lower airway inflammation. Since antileukotrienes have been shown to be beneficial to patients with aspirin-sensitive asthma, further studies are also required to ascertain their role in patients with aspirin sensitivity, allergic rhinitis and nasal polyposis.

Allergen avoidance

Frequently overlooked in the management of allergic and nonallergic rhinitis is the avoidance of allergens or irritants. Although common sense dictates that patients should be able to recognize causative factors in their rhinitis, re-enforcement by their physician can help in acknowledging avoidance techniques. In industrialized countries, most of an individual's personal time is spent indoors and this environment contains important triggers of rhinitis. The outdoor and indoor allergic and nonallergic environment has changed within the past 30 years and this has

Table 3.8
Intranasal medications for use in the treatment of allergic rhinitis.

	Drug	Trade name (dose/spray)	Daily dose/nostril	Paediatric indication
Antihistamines	Azelastine	Rhinolast (140 µg)	1 spray b.d.	≥5 years
	Levocabastine	Livostin (0.05%)	2 sprays b.d. max. 4 weeks	≥9 years
Corticosteroids	Beclomethasone	Beconase (50 µg)	2 sprays b.d. or 1 spray 3–4 times daily	≥6 years
	Budesonide	Beclomethasone (50 µg)	2 sprays b.d.	≥12 years
		Rhinocort Aqua (100 µg)	1–2 sprays b.d.	≥12 years
	Fluticasone	Flixonase (50 µg)	2 sprays o.d.–b.d.	4–11 years
			1 spray o.d.–b.d.	≥12 years
	Mometasone	Nasonex (50 µg)	2 sprays (4 max.) o.d.	≥12 years
	Dexamethasone	Dexa-Rhinaspray (20 µg)	1 spray 2–3 times daily (max. 4 days)	5–12 years
	Triamcinolone	Nasacort (55 µg)	1 spray b.d.	≥12 years
			2 sprays o.d.	
			1 spray o.d. (maintenance)	
	Flunisolide	Syntaris (25 µg)	1 spray o.d.	6–12 years
			2 sprays b.d.	≥12 years
Cromones	Cromoglycate	Rynacrom (4%)	1 squeeze 2–4 times daily	≥12 years
		Vividrin (2%)	1 spray 4–6 times daily	
	Nedocromil	Tilarin (1%)	1 spray 4 times daily	≥12 years
Anticholinergics	Ipratropium bromide	Rinatec (0.03% – 42 µg/dose) Atrovent	2 sprays 2–3 times daily	≥6 years

b.d. = twice daily; o.d. = once daily.

probably increased the risks and prevalence of allergic disease. Energy-saving building techniques have led to airtight houses with low natural ventilation and, subsequently, increased numbers of mites.

When possible, environmental control measures for indoor allergens should be applied even if their efficacy is not complete as they generally improve the patient's symptoms and reduce the need for pharmacological treatment. Furthermore, even when an allergic source (such as pets) is removed from a patient's environment, the benefit may take several weeks or months to be noticed. House dust mites and moulds thrive in high humidity and the scales of human skin are the main source of nutrition for dust mites. Nonspecific triggers, such as tobacco smoke, household chemicals and indoor pollution, should be avoided. Most of the avoidance measures should be concentrated initially in the patient's bedroom and, once completed, the common areas of the house should be dealt with next. It is usually helpful to provide patients with detailed written information; patient information leaflets are widely available for this purpose. Such guidance, in most instances, reduces the level of pharmacological treatment.

For patients who are pollen allergic, avoiding outdoor activities during peak pollination periods and keeping doors and windows closed during the spring and autumn pollen periods will help. Patients who are dust-mite allergic benefit by avoiding feather products, from the use of zippered vinyl encasements for their mattress and box spring, and from avoiding lying on carpeted surfaces. Common environmental measures for various allergic triggers are listed in Appendix I.

Immunotherapy

Desensitization with specific vaccines should be considered for patients with intractable symptoms, despite optimal environmental controls and conventional pharmacotherapy. The indications for specific desensitization immunotherapy are listed below (for more details, see Chapter 10):

- Failure to respond to a combination of proper allergen avoidance measures and pharmacotherapy.
- Severe persistent nasal or ocular symptoms.
- Prolonged seasonal allergy symptoms, such as symptoms lasting for 4–6 months for more than 2 years.
- A frequent need for systemic steroids to control allergy symptoms.

- Special situations in which allergen exposure cannot be avoided, such as veterinary physicians who have allergic rhinitis when exposed to animals.

Table 3.9 summarizes the pharmacotherapy of allergic rhinitis, and *Figure 3.2* illustrates a systematic approach to its management.

Management of allergic rhinitis in pregnancy

Allergic rhinitis affects approximately one third of women of child-bearing age and, hence, encountering this disorder during pregnancy is not uncommon. As with several other disorders, most pregnant women often experience an improvement in their symptoms from rhinitis due to the effects of placental hormones. There are, however, some women who still experience troublesome symptoms from rhinitis and who require pharmacotherapy. Most product labels of the agents used in allergic rhinitis state they should be avoided in pregnancy.

However, there are no controlled studies of pregnant women, and most of our knowledge in this area comes from research into electronic databases and other sources of information regarding the rate of foetal malformations in pregnant women treated with various agents for allergic rhinitis. Sodium cromoglycate and beclomethasone are used as first-line treatment in pregnancy. Beclomethasone has been used in the management of asthma during pregnancy without any untoward effects on the foetus. If the patient has already undergone a well established dose of immunotherapy, this

Table 3.9
Summary of medication efficacy on rhinitis symptoms.

	Sneezing	Discharge	Blockage	Anosmia
Cromoglycate	+ +	+	+	−
Decongestant	−	−	+ + +	−
Antihistamine	+ + +	+ +	+/ −	−
Ipratropium	−	+ +	−	−
Topical steroids	+ + +	+ +	+ +	+
Oral steroids	+ +	+ +	+ + +	+ +

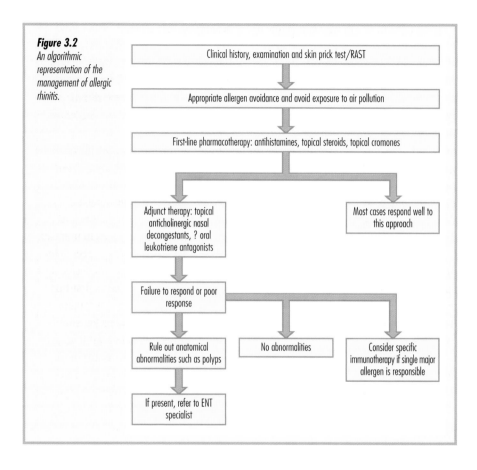

Figure 3.2
An algorithmic representation of the management of allergic rhinitis.

Clinical history, examination and skin prick test/RAST

↓

Appropriate allergen avoidance and avoid exposure to air pollution

↓

First-line pharmacotherapy: antihistamines, topical steroids, topical cromones

Adjunct therapy: topical anticholinergic nasal decongestants, ? oral leukotriene antagonists

Most cases respond well to this approach

Failure to respond or poor response

Rule out anatomical abnormalities such as polyps

No abnormalities

Consider specific immunotherapy if single major allergen is responsible

If present, refer to ENT specialist

can be continued since it does not seem to have any teratogenic effects. However, there is still a theoretical possibility of experiencing a systemic reaction and this should be discussed with the patient. If an antihistamine has to be used to alleviate the patient's symptoms, chlorpheniramine has been recommended based on its longevity and the more conclusive evidence of its safety.

Conclusion

Patients with allergic rhinitis feel their quality of life is worse compared with the general population. Allergic patients feel they have more fatigue, more physical limitations, decreased social functioning, increased pain and an overall poorer image compared with nonatopic patients and as measured by several surveys. Patients with rhiniti s also experience a significant perception of side-effects from their medication (31%), avoid drugs because of side-effects (65.1%) and worry about the side-effects of medication (48%). Patients frequently complain about decreased energy, possibly caused by the side-effects (sedation or insomnia as a result of the medication interfering with their sleep cycle). Headaches as a consequence of allergies usually result from hypertrophy of the turbinates or sinus inflammation. Some 46% of patients with rhinitis may have headaches, with discomfort to the frontal sinus distribution in 84% of patients. With the exceptions of sinusitis, food-induced migraines and discomfort to the frontal sinus distribution, the majority of headaches do not have an allergic origin and so other causes should be sought. Because of their perception of their poor health, some patients with chronic rhinitis may be refractory to standard treatments. Many of these patients have underlying psychological reasons for their complaints. When patients present with severe symptoms that are out of proportion to the objective evidence, that last longer than 6 months and are refractory to optimal medication and environmental controls, a diagnosis of undifferentiated somatoform disorder should be considered.

Appendix I: Environmental control measures

House dust mites
- Enclose the mattress, duvets and pillows with allergen-impermeable covers.
- Synthetic materials should be used in preference to down, wool or feathers.
- Vacuuming items of bedding, carpets, soft furnishings and curtains and washing these items at 60 °C at least once a week.
- Bedrooms should be damp-dusted weekly.
- Maintain indoor humidity at less than 40%.

Pets
- No hypoallergenic dog or cat breeds have been identified.
- Remove the pet (ideal).
- Wash the pet once a week (if it is not possible to remove the pet).
- No pets in the bedroom at any time.

Moulds

- Avoid damp, musty basements.
- In areas of high humidity, a dehumidifier can help.
- Avoid activities (e.g. raking leaves) that increase exposure to moulds.
- House plants should be kept to a minimum.
- Fungicides can be applied to surfaces with obvious contamination.
- Avoid live Christmas trees.

Pollens

- Monitor pollen forecasts and avoid high pollen areas.
- Keep windows closed in the house and car.
- Avoid activities that increase pollen exposure, such as mowing the lawn.
- Use an air conditioner.

Acknowledgements

The authors are grateful to Dr Dimitris Kasimos, Specialist Registrar in Paediatrics, for his help with this chapter.

Further reading

AAAAI Board of Directors. Position statement: guidelines to minimize the risk from systemic reaction caused by immunotherapy with allergic extracts. *J Allergy Clin Immunol* (1994) **93**: 811–12.

Bousquet J, Lebel B, Chanal I, Morel A, Michel FB. Antiallergic activity of H_1-receptor antagonists assessed by nasal challenge. *J Allergy Clin Immunol* (1988) **82**: 881–87.

Day James MD. Pros and cons of the use of antihistamines in managing allergic rhinitis. *J Allergy Clin Immunol* (1999) **103**: S395–99.

Druce HD. Allergic and nonallergic rhinitis. In: Middleton E, Reed CE, Ellis EF et al., eds. *Allergy: Principles and Practice* (4th edn) (Mosby-Year Book Co., St Louis, MO, 1993): 1433–53.

Howarth PH. Allergic rhinitis: a rational choice of treatment. *Respir Med* (1989) **83**: 179–88.

International Consensus Report (ICR) on diagnosis and management of rhinitis. *Allergy* (1994) **19**: 5–34.

International Consensus Report (ICR) on the diagnosis and management of rhinitis. *Allergy* (1994) **49**: 1–36.

Jacobs RL, Freedman PM, Boswell RN. Non-allergic rhinitis with eosinophilia (NARES syndrome): clinical and immunological presentation. *J Allergy Clin Immunol* (1981) **67**: 253–62.

Levenson T, Greenberger P. Pathophysiology and therapy for allergic and nonallergic rhinitis: an updated review. *Allergy Asthma Proc* (1997) **18:** 213–20.

Lierl M. Allergy of the upper respiratory tract. In: Lawlor G, Fisher T, Adelman D, eds. *Manual of Allergy and Immunology* (3rd edn) (Little, Brown & Co., Boston, MA, 1994): 94–111.

Lund V. Allergic rhinitis – making the correct diagnosis. *Clin Exp Allergy* (1998) **28 (suppl 6):** 25–28.

Mazzotta P, Loebstein R, Koren G. Treating allergic rhinitis in pregnancy. Safety considerations. *Drug Saf* (1999) **20:** 361–75.

Meltzer EO. An overview of current pharmacotherapy in perennial rhinitis. *J Allergy Clin Immunol* (1995) **95:** 1097–110.

Mullarkey M, Hill J, Webb D. Allergic and nonallergic rhinitis: their characterization with attention to the meaning of nasal eosinophilia. *J Allergy Clin Immunol* (1980) **65:** 122–26.

Norman PS. Allergic rhinitis. *J Allergy Clin Immunol* (1985) **75:** 531–48.

Peterson B, Saxon A. Global increases in allergic respiratory disease: the possible role of diesel exhaust particles. *Ann Allergy Asthma Immunol* (1996) **77:** 263–70.

Rachelefsky GS. Pharmacologic management of allergic rhinitis. *J Allergy Clin Immunol* (1998) **101:** 367–69.

Raphael GD, Hauptschein-Raphael M, Kaliner M. Gustatory rhinitis: a syndrome of food-induced rhinorrhea. *J Allergy Clin Immunol* (1989) **83:** 110–13.

Rupp GH, Friedman RA. Eosinophilic nonallergic rhinitis in children. *Pediatrics* (1982) **70:** 437–39.

Schalz M, Petitti D. Antihistamines and pregnancy. *Ann Allergy Asthma Immunol* (1997) **78:** 17–159.

Schuller D, Cadman T, Jeffreys W. Recurrent headaches: what every allergist should know. *Ann Allergy Asthma Immunol* (1996) **76:** 219–30.

Sibbald B, Rink E. Epidemiology of seasonal and perennial rhinitis: clinical presentation and medical history. *Thorax* (1991) **46:** 859–901.

Simons E. New medications for rhinitis. In: Busse W, Holgate S, eds. *Asthma and Rhinitis* (Blackwell, Cambridge, MA, 1995): 1325–36.

Simons FER, Simons KJ. The pharmacology and use of H1-receptor-antagonist drugs. *N Engl J Med* (1994) **330:** 1663–70.

Slavin RG. Nasal polyps and sinusitis. In: Middleton E Jr, Reed CE, Ellis EF et al., eds. *Allergy Principles and Practice* (4th edn) (Mosby-Year Book Co., St Louis, MO, 1993): 1455–70.

Storms W, Meltzer E, Nathan P, Selner I. Allergic rhinitis: the patient's perspective. *J Allergy Clin Immunol* (1997) **99:** 825–28.

Togias A, Naclerio PM, Proud D et al. Studies on the allergic and nonallergic inflammation. *J Allergy Clin Immunol* (1988) **81:** 782–90.

Wright AL, Holberg CJ, Martinez FD et al. Epidemiology of physician-diagnosed allergic rhinitis in childhood. *Pediatrics* (1994) **94:** 895–901.

Urticaria and angioedema

4

URTICARIA

Introduction

Urticaria (from the Latin *urtica* = a nettle) was described by Heberden in 1772 as:

> *the little elevations upon the skin ('nettle' rash) often appearing involuntarily, especially if the skin be rubbed, or scrubbed, and seldom staying many hours in the same place, and sometimes not many minutes. There is no body exempt from 'them' and by far the greatest number experience no other evil from it besides the intolerable anguish arising from the itching.*

Urticaria, commonly known as hives or wheals, is characterized by the appearance of erythematous, circumscribed, pruritic, occasionally burning or painful, cutaneous wheals. The skin lesions are raised plaques of regular or irregular border (annular urticaria). Individual lesions last for minutes to hours.

The entire process may occur over days or weeks. Urticaria present for fewer than 6 weeks is considered to be acute and episodes of urticaria lasting more than 6 weeks are classified as chronic. Urticaria is a common disorder and 15–25% of the general population will develop at least one such episode in their lives. Furthermore, chronic urticaria persists for at least one year in more than 50% of those affected, and for more than 20 years in 25% of those affected. Although urticaria appears in all age groups, acute urticaria is more common among children and young adults, whereas chronic urticaria occurs more often in adults, especially middle-aged women.

Urticaria can sometimes be accompanied by angioedema, which is typically described as the same process in the softer tissues of the face or throat but, on a pathologic basis, involves deeper dermal reactivity as well. Approximately half of the patients have urticaria with angioedema, 40% have pure urticaria and 10% have pure angioedema.

The primary physician's role includes searching for precipitants and underlying causes. Eliciting the cause can be difficult and is not always possible. The treatment of patients with chronic urticaria can present a significant challenge to the most experienced physician. It is not a single disease but a cutaneous reaction pattern for which there are multiple potential causes. The clinical expression of this disease varies from patient to patient, as do its duration of activity, the morphologic features of the lesions and its histopathologic basis.

Pathophysiology

Urticaria results from increased vascular permeability leading to extravasation of protein-rich fluid from small blood vessels, usually postcapillary venules. The localized accumulation of fluid produces the characteristic oedematous, erythematous papules, which are pruritic, blanch on pressure and range in size from a few millimetres to several centimetres, often with serpignious borders. Individual lesions rarely persist for longer than 24–48 hours, and often resolve sooner.

In angioedema, the extravasation of fluid occurs in deeper layers of the skin, showing a preference for the periorbital, perioral, palmar and plantar surfaces of the body. The oedema is more diffuse, and the overlying skin appears normal and does not itch.

Classification

Acute urticaria is extremely common, possibly affecting as many as 10–20% of the population at some time in their lives. It is most frequently a self-limited disorder caused by an allergic reaction to a food or drug. When the urticaria exceeds 6 weeks, it is rather arbitrarily designated as chronic. Different types of classification have been suggested, depending on pathophysiology, aetiology and clinical features. The classification given in **Table 4.1** is intended to provide a better understanding of urticaria with regard to its clinical evaluation and management.

Physical urticarias

The physical urticarias (**Table 4.2**) are a unique subgroup of chronic urticarias in which the wheals can usually be reproduced through the appropriate physical manoeuvres. Wheal formation is intermittent and occurs soon after the application of the stimulus (except in the case of delayed-pressure urticaria). The wheals have a distinctive appearance and location, and the eruption usually lasts less than 2 hours. Cold, heat, pressure, vibration, light, water, exercise and increases in core temperature have

all been demonstrated as provoking stimuli. Physical urticarias comprise up to 17% of chronic urticaria and occur more frequently in young adults. The physical urticarias are distinguished by the appearance of episodic lesions, often limited to the areas of inciting physical stimuli. In some patients, more than one type of physical urticaria may be present. There may also be systemic features, such as flushing, headaches, dizziness or hypotension. The urticarial lesions are at least in part due to mast cell activation and mediator release. However, the mechanism by which a physical stimulus to the skin releases mast cell mediators is not fully understood.

Infection

Urticaria may be a sign of viral, parasitic, bacterial or fungal infection. Eliminating a clinical infection in a patient with chronic urticaria may at times cause a decrease in the severity of the hives, but extremely rarely makes the hives disappear. Infections that have been associated with urticaria include streptococcal pharyngitis, otitis media, sinusitis, upper respiratory infections, mononucleosis, hepatitis, Coxsackie infections, mycoplasma infections, parasitic infections and fungal infections.

Table 4.1
The major causes of urticaria and angioedema that should be considered when any patient is being evaluated.

1 **Allergy**
Drug reactions
Food and food additives
Inhalation, ingestion of (or contact with)
antigens
Transfusion reactions
Insects (papular urticaria)

2 **Physical urticarias**
Dermographism
Solar urticaria
Cold urticaria
Localized heat urticaria; pressure
urticaria (angioedema)
Aquagenic urticaria
Cholinergic urticaria
Exercise-induced anaphylactic
syndrome
Delayed pressure urticaria/angioedema
Vibratory angioedema

3 **Hereditary diseases**
Hereditary angioedema
Familial cold urticaria
Hereditary vibratory angioedema
C3B inactivator deficiency
Muckel–Wells syndrome (amyloidosis
with deafness and urticaria)

4 **Infections**
Bacterial
Fungal
Viral
Helminthic

5 **Urticaria pigmentosa**
Systemic mastocytosis

6 **Immune complex diseases**
Urticarial vasculitis
Serum sickness
Systemic lupus erythematosis
Juvenile rheumatoid arthritis
Polyarteritis nodosa
Dermatomyositis
Neonatal lupus syndrome
Sjögren's syndrome
Rheumatic fever

7 **Malignancy**
Angioedema with acquired C1 and C1
inactivator (INH) depletion
Leukaemia
Lymphoma (Hodgkin's disease)
Myeloma
Carcinoma of colon, rectum, liver, lung
and ovary

8 **Endocrine disorders**
Diabetes mellitus
Hyperthyroidism
Hypothyroidism
Hyperparathyroidism
Ovarian hormonal effects

9 **Chronic idiopathic urticaria and
angioedema**

Table 4.2
Physical urticarias.

Dermographism
    Symptomatic
    Delayed
    White
    Cold-dependent

Solar urticaria

Cold urticaria   Primary/idiopathic cold urticaria
    Essential/acquired cold urticaria
    • Localized cold reflex urticaria
    • Systemic atypical acquired cold urticaria
    • Cold-dependent dermographism
    • Delayed cold urticaria
    • Cold-induced cholinergic urticaria
    • Cold erythema

    Familial cold urticaria
    • Immediate type
    • Late type

    Secondary/acquired
    • Mononucleosis
    • Connective tissue disease
    • Chronic lymphocytic leukaemia
    • Cryoglobulinaemia, cold agglutinins

Localized heat urticaria

Cholinergic urticaria

Exercise-induced anaphylactic syndrome

Aquagenic urticaria

Delayed-pressure urticaria/angioedema

Vibratory urticaria/angioedema
    Acquired
    Familial

Urticaria pigmentosa/mastocytosis

Mastocytosis is a disease whose clinical features include pruritus, urtication, flushing, nausea, diarrhoea, abdominal pain, vascular instability, headache and neuropsychiatric disorder problems. Mastocytosis can occur at any age and in several forms. The most common skin manifestation of mastocytosis in both children and adults is urticaria pigmentosa. Urticaria pigmentosa is observed in over 90% of patients with indolent mastocytosis but in fewer than 50% of patients with mastocytosis with an associated haematologic disorder or those with aggressive mastocytosis. Urticaria pigmentosa lesions appear as small, yellowish-tan to reddish-brown macules or slightly raised papules and, occasionally, as raised nodules or plaque-like lesions. The palms, soles, face and scalp tend to remain free of lesions. Scratching or rubbing of the lesions usually leads to urtication and erythema over and around the macules, known as Darier's sign. Urticaria pigmentosa is sometimes associated with pruritus that is often exacerbated by changes in temperature, local friction, the ingestion of hot beverages or spicy foods, ethanol and certain drugs.

H_1 and H_2 antihistamines have been used for its symptomatic treatment. Oral cromolyn sodium 100–200 mg q.i.d. has also proved effective in controlling gastrointestinal symptoms and in reducing the severity of attacks.

Urticarial vasculitis

Urticarial vasculitis is a disorder that presents clinically as an urticarial eruption but that histopathologically shows a picture of vasculitis. There are some diagnostically useful clinical differences between 'classical' urticaria and urticarial vasculitis. In urticarial vasculitis the lesions are present for a longer duration – often between 3 and 7 days. In contrast to the predominant symptom of itching in urticaria, patients with urticarial vasculitis also describe burning and, sometimes, painful lesions. Urticarial vasculitis may present as purpuric or frankly vasculitic lesions in addition to urticarial lesions and, rarely, bullae may occur. While clearing, the urticarial lesions may leave residual erythema, scaling or purpura. Urticarial vasculitis may also present as angioedema, which may also leave a residual, bruised appearance with scaling or purpura. Since treatment with H_1 antihistamines is generally ineffective in controlling symptoms, urticarial vasculitis should be considered in patients with apparently intractable urticaria who do not respond to antihistamines.

Patients with urticarial vasculitis frequently have associated fever, myalgias, arthralgias and sometimes arthritis, as well as leukocytosis and elevated sedimentation rate. Hypocomplementemic and normocomplementemic forms have been described. The incidence of systemic involvement in urticarial vasculitis follows the pattern of involvement in systemic vasculitis. Joint involvement occurs in up to 75% of patients, renal involvement in 30%, gastrointestinal involvement in 25%, pulmonary involvement in 20% and ophthalmic involvement in 10%. Joint problems may range from flitting arthalgia to full-blown arthritis. Microscopic haematuria and proteinuria are present if the kidneys are involved, but impairment of renal function is rare. Abdominal pain, nausea, vomiting and diarrhoea may occur, and pulmonary problems include chronic obstructive airway disease, asthma or pleural effusions. Neurological involvement may simulate a tumour or cause optic atrophy. Conjunctivitis, uveitis and episcleritis can occur.

Chronic idiopathic urticaria

Chronic urticaria is defined as the occurrence of widespread wheals daily (or almost daily) for at least 6 weeks. The term 'chronic idiopathic urticaria' is used where urticarial vasculitis and predominant physical urticarias have been excluded.

The exact incidence and prevalence of chronic idiopathic urticaria are not known, although it occurs in at least 0.1% of the population; it is twice as common in women as in men. Severe chronic idiopathic urticaria is a disabling condition and may be acutely distressing particularly when, as in 50% of cases, it occurs with angioedema. This produces sudden localized swellings of the skin and mucous membranes, which are especially unpleasant on the face, lips, tongue and in the respiratory tract, and which resolve spontaneously over a day or two. Chronic idiopathic urticaria has a chronic relapsing course and about 20% of patients still have it 10 years after first presentation. It may be difficult to treat, with poor response to conventional antihistamine therapy.

Recent studies have shown that up to 30% of cases of chronic urticarias are indeed of the autoimmune type. These patients have functional IgG anti-FcεR1 auto-antibodies. These antibodies bind to the α-peptide portion of FcεR1 and can directly cross-link to adjacent receptors leading to mast cell activation without the intervention of IgE. Skin prick tests (SPT) carried out with autologous serum from these patients show whealing responses in the uninvolved skin.

Dermatological illustrations of urticaria are shown in *Figures 4.1* and *4.2*.

An approach to a patient with urticaria

Chronic urticaria poses significant diagnostic and management challenges. Urticaria can be caused by a variety of exogenous factors, including drugs and chemicals, foods, cosmetics, physical stimuli and, less commonly, inhalants. Endogenous sources of urticaria include infections, infestations, endocrinopathies and certain systemic diseases (*Table 4.1*).

History

A detailed clinical history is of utmost importance in the evaluation of a patient with urticaria. If the history does not suggest a cause, it is most unlikely that any routine battery of tests would identify any occult cause. It is essential that both the physician and patient appreciate the fact that almost all the patients who present with hives for 4–6 weeks have idiopathic urticaria.

Inquiry into recent illness, medications, foods and inhalants that have been associated with urticaria may help to determine the proximate cause of the urticarial reaction. Patients should be encouraged to keep a food dairy and should be alerted to include such items as toothpaste, cosmetics, food additives and birth control pills. Agents that may be entering through the conjunctiva, nasal mucosa, rectum or vaginal area should not be overlooked. Information about intake of milk products and beer should be obtained, because penicillin in dairy products or yeast in beer can precipitate urticaria. Parasympathetic symptoms, such as abdominal cramps, diarrhoea, headache, salivation and diaphoresis, must be checked. It is important to determine whether exposure to pressure, cold, light, heat or exercise precipitates lesions. A travel history may suggest a parasitic infestation. Inquiry into agents and factors that might modulate the intensity of an urticarial reaction (e.g. aspirin, alcohol, NSAIDs (nonsteroidal anti-inflammatory drugs), heat, humidity, occlusive clothing, psychological stress) can provide clinically useful information. Questions pertaining to routine systemic inquiry are helpful in identifying an underlying systemic disease.

Figure 4.1
Urticarial lesions on the lower limb.

Source: Courtesy of Professor P Friedman, Department of Dermatology, University of Southampton.

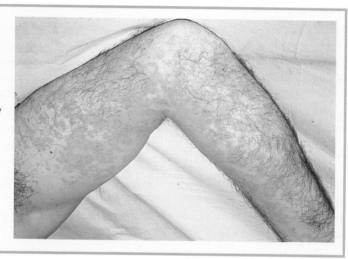

Figure 4.2
Giant urticaria on the thigh.

Source: Courtesy of Professor P Friedman, Department of Dermatology, University of Southampton.

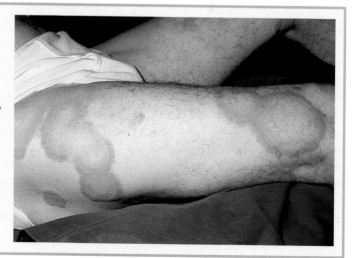

Physical examination

Dermatographism is associated with linear wheals. Small lesions with erythematous flares are typical of cholinergic urticaria. Periorbital or perioral swelling is suggestive of angioedema. Careful examination of the ears, pharynx, sinuses and teeth may help uncover a focal infection. Lymphadenopathy and hepatosplenomegaly are suggestive of an underlying lymphoma or hepatocellular disease. The joints are noted for swelling, effusion and warmth, which are suggestive of active rheumatoid disease.

Laboratory studies

It is usually unproductive to attempt a diagnosis through the performance of an extensive panel of laboratory tests in the absence of positive evidence from a clinical history, suggestive of historic and physical examination. An initial laboratory evaluation of a patient for chronic urticaria should include a complete haemogram with a differential and platelet count, an assessment of erythrocyte sedimentation rate (ESR), an antinuclear antibody analysis, liver enzyme analysis and urinalysis. Skin prick tests (SPT) and radio allergosorbent testing (RAST) have minimal value. Complement levels, including C4, C3 and C1-esterase inhibitor (INH), are

performed to rule out hereditary angioedema (HAE). Skin biopsy is usually not necessary to diagnose urticaria but should be considered if vasculitis is suspected. Stool examination for ova and parasites is appropriate if recent diarrhoeal illness or travel to endemic areas have taken place. A complete list of the investigations that could be useful in the assessment of urticaria is given in **Table 4.3**, but in routine practice most of these tests are not performed.

Provocative testing of physical urticarias

The following tests can be performed:

- *Dermatographism* Stroke the skin with a dermatographometer at 3600 g/cm^2.
- *Cholinergic* Exercise or a warm bath to raise core temperature by 0.7–1.0 °C. Methacholine skin test: intradermal injection of methacholine, 0.1 ml of a 1:500 dilution.
- *Localized heat* Apply a heated cylinder (50–55 °C) to the skin for 5 minutes.
- *Solar* Perform phototesting with ultraviolet and fluorescent light.
- *Aquagenic* Apply water compresses (35 °C) to the skin of the upper body for 30 minutes.
- *Vibratory* Apply vortex vibration to the forearm for 5 minutes.

Table 4.3
Laboratory investigations in urticaria/angioedema.

Full blood count
ESR
Blood sugar
Liver function tests
Urea and electrolytes, serum alanine transferase
Urinalysis
Hepatitis serology
Serum total IgE
Skin prick tests
RAST
Rheumatoid factor
C1 esterase inhibitor absolute amount and functional assay activation
C_1q, C_2, C_3, C_4 complement factors
Cryoglobulins
Autoimmune profile
Chest X-ray

- *Delayed pressure* Apply a 7.5 Kg weight to the skin for 20 minutes with inspection at 4–8 hours.
- *Primary cold* Apply a plastic-wrapped ice cube to the skin for 4 minutes.
- *Familial cold* Expose to cold air for 20–30 minutes (ice cube test results are negative).

Management

The first rule in managing patients with urticaria is to avoid or to remove the inciting trigger. Therapy is aimed at providing symptomatic relief rather than suppressing the urticaria. Initially, it is important to reassure the patient that, although urticaria is bothersome and in some situations a worrisome condition, it is benign. An exception is in the case of angioedema, where life-threatening airway compromise can be a consequence. Aside from the avoidance of triggering agents, the mainstay of treatment is with antihistamines.

Chronic urticaria varies clinically and histopathologically. The origin of acute urticaria can be detected in some cases but in patients with chronic urticaria the cause is rarely identified. Thus, most patients with chronic urticaria are considered to have idiopathic disease. The natural history of chronic idiopathic urticaria is described as the duration of each continuous episode:

- 50% resolve spontaneously in 3–12 months.
- 20% resolve spontaneously in 12–36 months.
- 20% resolve spontaneously in 36–60 months.
- 1.5% last 20–25 years.

When angioedema accompanies the urticaria, 75% of patients have symptoms for more than 1 year and 20% for more than 20 years. The algorithmic clinical approach to the management of urticaria is shown in *Figure 4.3*.

Pharmacotherapy

Antihistamines

Antihistamines are the mainstay of therapy for both acute and chronic urticaria and angioedema. Histamine antagonists (H_1 and H_2 type) are highly selective and compete peripherally with histamine for their respective receptor sites. The binding at the receptor site is reversible both for the histamine and the antagonist. The binding of the histamine to its H_1 receptor lasts from 15 minutes to 24 hours, and antihistamines do not displace histamine that is already bound but will delay activation of the receptor by histamine. Therefore, the best results are achieved by having antihistamines on the receptors before the histamine arrives and then maintaining them 'round the clock'. Antihistamines do not always decrease the number of urticarial lesions or the frequency of eruptions, but they significantly diminish pruritus.

The choice of antihistamine to be used is based on its effectiveness, frequency of administration and its side-effects profile. The dose of the H_1 antagonist should be increased to tolerance. Most of the first-generation antihistamines are equivalent in effectiveness, with the major difference usually being the degree of sedation or anticholinergic effect they produce. If a first-generation antihistamine is well tolerated, it should be preferred because it is usually as effective as the nonsedating antihistamines and is much less expensive.

There are situations, however, in which first-generation antihistamines alone do not seem to control the urticaria. In such cases a combination of two non-

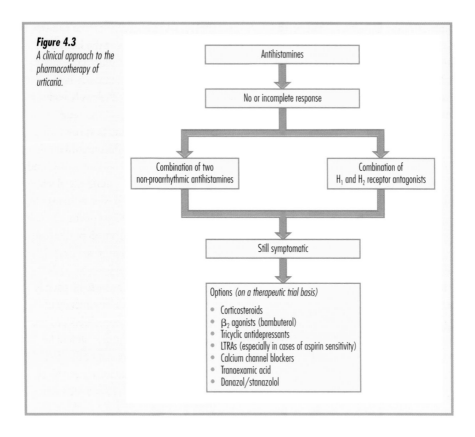

Figure 4.3
A clinical approach to the pharmacotherapy of urticaria.

proarrhythmic antihistamines can be used. One approach is to use a nonsedating (daytime) antihistamine alongside a sedating antihistamine (evening). Patients can sometimes tolerate the side-effects of one antihistamine better than those of another, even though the doses used are comparable. Therefore, different preparations (even from the same category) should be tried.

If adequate relief is not achieved at the maximal tolerated dose, H_2 antagonists cimetidine 300 mg 4 times a day or ranitidine 150 mg twice a day may be added. H_2 antagonists can be effective, especially if the patient demonstrates dermographism or flushing with the urticaria. The rationale is that the cutaneous vasculature possesses not only a large number of H_1 receptors but also a small number of H_2 receptors.

Once the H_1 receptors have been blocked, the addition of an antihistamine that binds to H_2 receptors augments the antihistamine effect. The use of an H_2-receptor antagonist alone has no effect on urticaria and, on the contrary, H_2 blockers may counteract the normal feedback inhibition of histamine on mast cell degranulation and thus act counterproductively. Hence, H_2 antagonists should be used in combination with other medications and never as a sole regimen. Unless their use has clearly improved the urticaria, discontinuation of H_2 blockers within 3 weeks is recommended.

Another approach is to use triple therapy with the nonsedating and somewhat sedating antihistamines, as well as a short course of prednisone to induce remission. Subsequently, one may continue the antihistamines for several weeks after the hives have disappeared before removing those drugs on a slow, tapering schedule. The rationale behind this approach is that the reactivity of the mast cell or the other neuroimmunologic factors that were activated becomes quiescent and controlled, and so the blocking agents can be withdrawn. Patients are urged to keep a supply of the antihistamines available so that at the first sign of a recurrence of the urticaria they may initiate therapy again.

Corticosteroids

Glucocorticoids are indicated for their anti-inflammatory and immunosuppressant effects. They provide symptomatic relief and have no effect on the underlying disease process. The use of corticosteroids does not eliminate the need for other therapies. Their immunosuppressant action prevents or suppresses cell-mediated immune reactions, reducing the accumulation of T-cells, monocytes and eosinophils. They have no place as regular therapy in chronic urticaria, although they may be administered as a pulse dose to break the cycle of a resistant episode. Corticosteroids in patients with chronic urticaria are used when the symptoms are unresponsive to antihistamines as used in maximal dosage and the symptoms are disabling in terms of functioning at home or in the workplace. Although skin biopsies of chronic urticaria are considered unrewarding, they are of value in some patients who are not responding to treatment, prior to starting corticosteroids.

Leukotriene receptor antagonists (LTRAs)

A subset of patients with chronic urticaria experience improved control using leukotriene antagonists. In patients with chronic urticaria, the prevalence of sensitivity to aspirin and nonsteroidal anti-inflammatory drugs is estimated to be between 21 and 30%. The pathogenesis of aspirin sensitivity most likely involves inhibition of cyclo-oxygenase by aspirin or nonsteroidal anti-inflammatory drugs, resulting in a change in the balance of arachidonic acid metabolites and an increase in leukotriene LTB_4, LTC_4, LTD_4 and LTE_4. Because of this imbalance, patients with aspirin sensitivity and chronic urticaria may be more likely to respond to leukotriene antagonists than those lacking this sensitivity. The addition of montelukast 10 mg/d or zafirlukast 20 mg twice daily has been shown to achieve control in patients who have otherwise been unresponsive to antihistamines. Further research into the use of leukotriene antagonists in patients with chronic urticaria, particularly those with aspirin sensitivity, is warranted.

β_2 agonists

Beta agonists, such as bambuterol, may have an adjunct effect when used with other agents in patients with intractable urticaria as a result of their membrane-stabilizing action. Adverse effects such as tremors and palpitations may limit their use.

Table 4.4 lists all the drugs (and their doses) that can be used in urticaria.

Patient education

It is important to discuss with the patient that most chronic forms are idiopathic and that a cause may not be found. Emphasize the variable natural history of the hives and the high probability that lesions will disappear spontaneously. Prepare the patient for the likelihood that urticaria will recur. Instruct all patients to avoid definite provocative factors, if any, such as aspirin, heat, exertion and alcoholic beverages. Specific advice, such as the avoidance of swimming in cold water for patients with cold urticaria, can be lifesaving. Reassure the patient that the medical investigation will exclude serious and/or treatable diseases and that many options are available to shorten the process and to alleviate the symptoms.

Table 4.4
Pharmacotherapy of urticaria/angioedema.

Drug	Dosage (in adults)
First-generation antihistamines	
Chlorpheniramine	4 mg q.d.s.
Clemastine	1 mg b.d., up to 6 mg/d
Cyproheptadine	4 mg q.d.s.
Hydroxyzine	25 mg nocte, up to 25 mg q.d.s.
Promethazine	25 mg b.d.
Second-generation antihistamines	
Cetirizine	10 mg/d
Loratadine	10 mg/d
Fexofenadine	180 mg/d
Mizolastine	10 mg/d
Beta agonists	
Bambuterol	10–20 mg/d
LTRAs	
Montelukast	10 mg/d at bedtime
Zafirlukast	20 mg b.d.
Antifibrinolytics	
ε-amino caproic acid	7–10 g/d
Tranexamic acid	1–2 g/d
Anabolic steroids	
Stanazolol	2.5–10 mg/d
Danazol	50–400 mg/d

The reduction of unrealistic expectations can reduce the disappointment that may follow a negative inquiry. It is important to emphasize the overall good prognosis and the high probability that remission will occur but that it might be delayed.

ANGIOEDEMA

C1 esterase inhibitor (C1-INH) deficiency

Deficiency of C1-INH can result in recurrent episodes of angioedema, and this was first described by Osler in 1888. Notably, urticaria does not occur as a consequence of C1-INH deficiency. Two types of C1-INH deficiency and their subtypes have been described:

1 Acquired angioedema (AAE) Type I and II.
2 Hereditary angioedema (HAE) Type I and II.

AAE I has been reported in association with Waldenström's macroglobulinaemia and lymphoproliferative disorders. AAE II has been recently identified and is secondary to an auto-antibody directed against C1-INH, rendering it nonfunctional. These patients lack a family history of recurrent angioedema and the disorder presents after the fourth decade of life with a malignancy or autoimmune disease.

HAE I is a consequence of a change in the genomic sequence of the C1-INH gene, impairing an mRNA transcription and translation of functional C1-INH protein. HAE I accounts for more than 80% of cases of hereditary C1-INH deficiency. The prevalence of HAE I is 1:150 000. HAE II accounts for the remaining 15% of HAE and is a consequence of a change in the genomic sequence of the C1-INH gene, yielding a nonfunctional C1-INH protein.

Clinical features and diagnosis

Angioedema is the principal presenting feature of all cases of HAE and AAE. The severity can vary from mild, painless, nonpruritic swellings affecting the peripheral soft tissue of the face to life-threatening attacks causing asphyxiation due to involvement of the larynx or oropharynx. Rarely, intravascular volume depletion can be so severe secondary to extravasation of plasma that severe hypotension can occur. Gastrointestinal involvement can present as abdominal pain, vomiting, diarrhoea or intestinal obstruction, mimicking an acute surgical emergency. Involvement of the central nervous system (CNS) can lead to cerebral oedema, seizures or hemiparesis. Factors that can predispose to acute attacks include trauma, stress, infections, surgical procedures and menstruation.

Causes of angioedema are summarized in *Table 4.5* and typical patterns seen on serological testing for complements are shown in *Figure 4.4*. In cases of HAE, it would be wise to screen family members (other siblings in particular).

Management

Treatment of HAE

Acute attacks

Maintenance of the airways is most important. IV fluids are administered to maintain intravascular volume. Depending on the symptoms and the site of the angioedema, intubation and other

Table 4.5
The causes of angioedema.

1 **Allergic (IgE-mediated)**, i.e. food, drugs, stings, parasites, inhalants
2 **Idiopathic**
3 **Physical stimuli**, i.e. cold, sunlight, pressure, vibration
4 **Non-IgE-mediated drug-induced**
    Histamine releases, i.e. narcotics, radiocontrast media
    Aspirin and other NSAIDs
    Angiotensin-converting enzyme inhibitors
5 **Deficiency of C1 inhibitor**
    Hereditary angioedema Type I
    Hereditary angioedema Type II
    Acquired deficiency Type I
    Acquired deficiency Type II
6 **Possible circulating immune complexes**
    Serum sickness
    Systemic lupus erythematosis
    Urticarial vasculitis
7 **Miscellaneous syndromes**
    Cutaneous/systemic mastocytosis
    Facial angioedema and eosinophilia
    C3b inactivator deficiency
    Carboxy peptidase B deficiency
    Urticaria/angioedema, deafness and amyloidosis (Muckel–Wells syndrome)

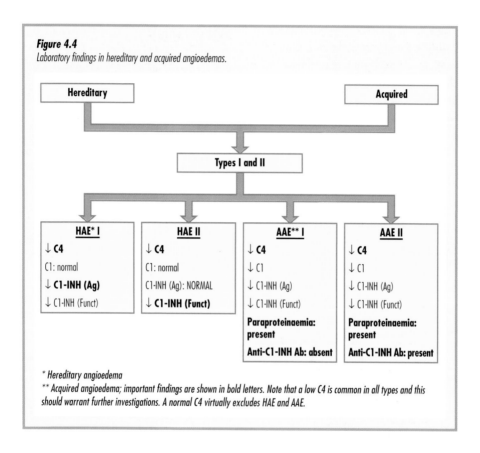

Figure 4.4
Laboratory findings in hereditary and acquired angioedemas.

HAE* I	HAE II	AAE** I	AAE II
↓ **C4**	↓ **C4**	↓ **C4**	↓ **C4**
C1: normal	C1: normal	↓ C1	↓ C1
↓ **C1-INH (Ag)**	C1-INH (Ag): NORMAL	↓ C1-INH (Ag)	↓ C1-INH (Ag)
↓ C1-INH (Funct)	↓ **C1-INH (Funct)**	↓ C1-INH (Funct)	↓ C1-INH (Funct)
		Paraproteinaemia: present	**Paraproteinaemia: present**
		Anti-C1-INH Ab: absent	**Anti-C1-INH Ab: present**

Hereditary angioedema
**Acquired angioedema; important findings are shown in bold letters. Note that a low C4 is common in all types and this should warrant further investigations. A normal C4 virtually excludes HAE and AAE.*

intensive support may be necessary. An acute attack that threatens airway obstruction should be treated with intramuscular epinephrine (0.3–0.5 ml of 1:1000). Patients with known angioedema should carry an epinephrine self-injection. In cases of gastrointestinal involvement narcotics are given to control the pain and nasogastric suction may be required to control emesis.

In HAE the treatment of choice in acute attacks consists of replacement therapy with commercially available, purified, vapour-treated C1-INH concentrates or, less preferentially, with fresh-frozen plasma. Administration of C1-INH concentrate in a dose of 500–1000 units by IV infusion will begin to resolve the angioedema within 30 minutes to 2 hours, with complete remission by 24 hours (1 unit is equivalent to C1 esterase activity of 1 ml of normal plasma). The clinical effect of this effusion lasts 3–5 days. Vapour-heated C1-INH concentrate inactivates hepatitis virus and HIV, both of which have been reported to be transmitted with purified C1-INH from human plasma.

Maintenance therapy

Attenuated anabolic steroids   The best treatment is the prevention of attacks, especially if they are frequent or severe (or both). Androgens have an anabolic effect on the production of C1-INH alleles, thereby causing increased synthesis of the protein and restored levels of C1-INH and C4. Attenuated androgens, including danazol or stanazolol, are widely used (for the dosage, see *Table 4.4*). It is important that treatment should be directed by clinical response and not by laboratory values. The masculizing effects of attenuated androgens are minimal at the dosage used, and only seldom do they affect menstruation. Liver function should be monitored periodically. Androgen use is not generally recommended in children unless attacks are severe and frequent, and should be instituted only after consultation with an endocrinologist. In both adults and children, weekly purified C1-INH concentrates can be used to prevent acute attacks.

Antifibrinolytics   ε-amino caproic acid or tranexamic acid has been used successfully to prevent acute attacks in HAE. They are competitive inhibitors of plasminogen activation and plasmin activity. Although they do not correct the serological abnormalities, they have been shown to be useful for maintenance therapy. Side-effects (including myonecrosis and vascular thrombosis) have diminished their use in favour of attenuated androgens. If used, it is recommended that antifibrinolytics be discontinued prior to major surgical procedures in view of the risk of thrombosis, and alternative prophylactic measures should be instituted, such as C1-INH concentrate or attenuated androgens.

Preoperative prophylaxis

Short-term prophylactic therapy is indicated in the setting of impending surgical or dental procedures where local or general anaesthetics are to be used. In addition, such prophylaxis is also indicated prior to dental or diagnostic procedures, such as endoscopy or bronchoscopy. Various regimes have been used, and these are as follows:

- Stanozolol or danazol are the most widely used agents. The dosage can be temporarily increased in patients who are already on maintenance therapy.
- Effective prophylaxis can also be reliably accomplished with the use of two units of frozen plasma given the day before and again immediately before the procedure.
- Purified C1-INH concentrate (given at doses of 1000–2000 units 2 hours prior to surgery) has been reported to be effective in anecdotal cases.

HAE during pregnancy

There is no consensus on the management of HAE during pregnancy. Like most disorders, the frequency and severity of attacks often subside during pregnancy but, nevertheless, there will be patients whose condition might prove difficult to manage. In view of their virilizing effects on the foetus, androgens are contraindicated. The episodic use of antifibrinolytic drugs has been found to be useful in reducing the severity and length of attacks in case reports. Similarly, there are reports of the successful treatment of acute attacks with purified C1-INH concentrate. Prophylactic replacement with C1-INH concentrate is generally not recommended in normal vaginal deliveries, but has been successfully used before caesarian sections.

Treatment of AAE

The treatment of acute attacks of angioedema in AAE is similar to that of HAE. Higher doses of androgens may be required during maintenance therapy. The underlying malignancy should be treated effectively by surgery or chemotherapy, as the case may be, and this will reduce C1-INH consumption by the tumour mass.

To date, the only therapeutic intervention that may alleviate AAE II is immunosuppressive therapy to decrease auto-antibody production. Plasmapheresis with 5% human serum albumin replacement relieved patients of the antibody load and angioedema. Additional therapy with pulsed cyclophosphamide produced a sustained remission.

The impact on life of urticaria and angioedema

One of the outcomes of a chronic condition such as urticaria is interference with lifestyle. For many, the condition is an irritant. As seen in case studies, the individual learns what triggers the symptoms and he or she modifies his or her behaviour accordingly. Activities such as hiking or running may be impossible if they precipitate uncontrollable itching and hives for someone with cholinergic urticaria. Canoeing, rafting or swimming may be impossible for the individual with severe cold urticaria. For those whose symptoms are severe or life-threatening, the prospect of accidentally finding themselves in situations that produce the urticaria can be a major source of fear and anxiety.

Another issue affecting the life of a person with urticaria is the discovery that others do not understand (or have not heard of) the condition. Many health care providers are not familiar with, and do not screen for, the physical urticarias. In the larger picture of overall health care, these problems are often dismissed as minor annoyances, without due consideration for diagnosis and treatment. However, worse than the health care provider's lack of interest and knowledge may be the response of the individual's family, friends or acquaintances, who are likely to be much less aware of the condition than health care providers.

As is the case with other conditions about which little is known, it can be difficult for health care providers to help a person whose symptoms do not fit into a recognizable framework. If there is not a familiar explanation or ready diagnosis, it is often too easy for a health care provider, as well as a lay person, to dismiss the symptoms and the impact they may have on someone's life. On the other hand, the majority of cases are destined to remain in the area of 'idiopathic urticaria'.

Further reading

Casale TB, Sampson MA, Hanifin J et al. The Cutaneous Allergy Committee, American Academy of Allergy and Immunology. Guide to physical urticarias. *J Allergy Clin Immunol* (1988) **82**: 758–63.

Ellis MH. Successful treatment of chronic urticaria with leukotriene antagonists. *J Allergy Clin Immunol* (1998) **102**: 876–7.

Heymann WR. Acquired angioedema. *J Am Acad Dermatol* (1997) **36**: 611–15.

Heymann WR. Chronic urticaria and angioedema associated with thyroid autoimmunity: review and therapeutic implications. *J Am Acad Dermatol* (1999) **40**: 229–32.

Kennedy MS. Comprehensive care in the allergy/asthma office: evaluation of chronic eczema and urticaria and angioedema. *Immunol Allergy Clin North Am* (1999) **19:** 19–33.

Kulp-Shorten CL, Callen JP. Clinical immunology and the rheumatologist: urticaria, angioedema, and rheumatologic disease. *Rheum Dis Clin North Am* (1996) **2:** 95–115.

Tharp MD. Risk management in asthma and allergic disease – chronic urticaria: pathophysiology and treatment approaches. *J Allergy Clin Immunol* (1996) **98:** 325–30.

Thiers BH, Beltrani VS. Urticaria and angioedema. *Curr Therapy Dermatologic Clinics* (1996) **14:** 171–98.

Tong LJ, Balakrishnan G. Clinical aspects of allergic disease: assessment of autoimmunity in patients with chronic urticaria. *J Allergy Clin Immunol* (1997) **99:** 461–5.

Weston WL, Badgett JT. Urticaria. *Pediat Rev* (1998) **19:** 240–4.

Zacharisen MC. Pediatric allergy and pediatric immunology: urticaria and angioedema. *Immunol Allergy Clin North Am* (1999) **19:** 363–82.

Anaphylaxis

5

Introduction

Anaphylaxis is a severe systemic allergic reaction mediated by interaction between the allergen, specific IgE antibody directed against this allergen and the high-affinity receptor on the surface of the mast cells and basophils. This process results in degranulation of the mast cell/basophil followed by release of vasoactive mediators into the circulation, causing a generalized reaction. However, there are instances when mast cells can be activated by non-IgE-dependent mechanisms, such as via activation of the complement or arachidonate pathways or even by a direct cellular activation. Such systemic reactions occurring via non-IgE-dependent mechanisms are referred to as 'anaphylactoid reactions'.

Data regarding the incidence of anaphylactic reactions are limited. Although asthmatics are at a greater risk of a fatal outcome in a severe reaction, the atopic status *per se* does not put them at a higher risk. Approximately 40 deaths per year in the USA are thought to result from

Hymenoptera stings. However, the risk of nonfatal anaphylaxis from Hymenoptera stings has been reported to be <1%. Whilst fatal anaphylaxis from penicillin allergy has been estimated to have an incidence of 0.002%, the risk of nonfatal anaphylaxis may range from 0.7 to 10%. In a study carried out in the UK, the incidence of severe anaphylaxis presenting as loss of consciousness or collapse in the emergency room has been estimated to be equivalent to 1 in 10 000 of the population per year.

Pathogenesis

In the case of IgE-mediated reactions, *prior* sensitization to the allergen is necessary. Upon subsequent exposure to even a minute quantity of the offending substance, the antigen or the allergen cross-links with the high-affinity FcεR1 receptor on the surface of the mast cell or basophil and induces degranulation and release of preformed and newly formed mediators (histamine, prostaglandin D_2 and tryptase) that are responsible for the reaction. These mediators induce smooth muscle contraction, vasodilatation and increased capillary permeability, and also cause chemotaxis of other inflammatory cells. In some cases, the allergen/antigen binds covalently to a low molecular protein (hapten) and the specific IgE is directed against this complex. In cases of non-IgE-mediated reaction, the activation of mast cells occurs via the formation of immune complexes, the activation of complement or coagulation pathways or it is kinin-mediated. *Figure 5.1* summarizes the various agents known to induce anaphylactic reactions together with their underlying mechanisms.

Clinical features

Onset of the reaction is usually within a few seconds or minutes following exposure to the allergen. Early symptoms include generalized pruritus, a tingling sensation in the hands, feet, lips and oropharynx, an impending sense of doom or catastrophe, dizziness, light-headedness, abdominal cramps, nausea and vomiting. In some cases a full-blown reaction may be preceded by generalized urticaria. In the case of patients who develop laryngeal oedema, a sensation of tingling and constriction in the throat is followed rapidly by a choking sensation. In lower airway involvement, cough, dyspnoea and wheeze are common. When the cardiovascular system is involved, patients experience chest pain, palpitations and syncope. Some cases are complicated by myocardial infarction and seizures. Twenty per cent of patients will develop

Figure 5.1
Agents causing anaphylaxis and their underlying mechanisms.

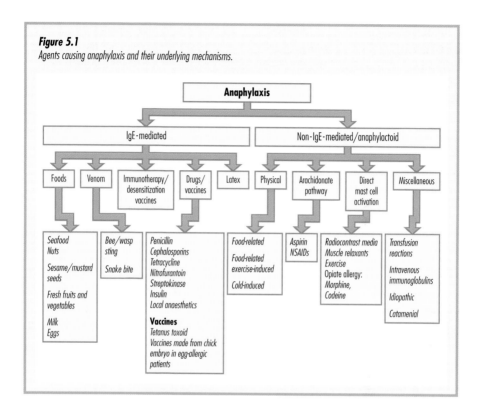

further symptoms up to 8 hours following resolution of the initial symptoms–biphasic reaction.

Differential diagnosis

Diagnosis is usually straightforward. However, in certain situations there may be some doubt when an anaphylactic reaction has to be distinguished from other conditions.

Vasovagal attack

In a vasovagal attack there is usually pallor as opposed to the flushing seen in anaphylaxis. In addition, in a vasovagal attack, hypotension is associated with bradycardia and not tachycardia, which is a feature of anaphylaxis. In a vasovagal attack, the symptoms are relieved rapidly by lying the patient flat.

Mastocytosis

This condition is characterized by a localized (mastocytoma) or generalized proliferation of mast cells. Patients have recurrent attacks of flushing, urticaria, nasal and gastrointestinal symptoms. Upper airway obstruction does not occur, and bronchospasm is unusual but, if it does occur, is usually transient. Patients usually have skin involvement in the form of urticaria pigmentosa and mast cell hyperplasia is often demonstrable in the affected organs, including the skin, the gastrointestinal tract and bone marrow. Elevated plasma histamine and serum tryptase can occur in mastocytosis as well as in anaphylaxis.

Cold-induced urticaria and cholinergic urticaria

These disorders are precipitated by exposure to cold temperatures or extreme changes in temperature, respectively. In an emergency situation it may be extremely difficult to differentiate them from anaphylaxis. Diagnosis of cold-induced urticaria is often made from the patient's history and via the 'ice cube test'. Similarly, cholinergic urticaria is diagnosed from the patient's history and by performing passive heat challenges.

There have been several reports of recurrent episodes of anaphylaxis in certain patients for no apparent reason. These patients usually present with episodes of flushing, tachycardia, angioedema, urticaria, upper airway obstruction, broncospasm, hypotension and syncope. Diagnosis is based on clinical signs and symptoms, raised serum tryptase, urinary histamine and the exclusion of other causes. This condition is known as recurrent idiopathic anaphylaxis.

Some patients develop anaphylaxis after undertaking physical exercise (exercise-induced anaphylaxis) or after ingesting a specific food followed immediately by physical exercise (food-related exercise-induced anaphylaxis). In the latter condition, specific IgE to the respective food is often demonstrable. Another rare syndrome that has been described is catamenial anaphylaxis. Patients experience recurrent cyclical episodes that coincide with the luteal phase of the menstrual cycle and, indeed, skin prick testing (SPT) demonstrates positive reactions to medroxyprogesterone. These patients also experience systemic reactions to luteinizing hormone-releasing hormone (LHRH) infusions and respond to ovarian suppression with LHRH agonists or oopherectomy.

Laboratory investigations

Tryptase (a product specific for mast cells) can be shown to be elevated in the sera of patients from 2–3 hours after onset of the symptoms and up to 6 hours afterwards. Other nonspecific abnormalities (such as elevation in serum and urinary methyl-histamine, in immune complexes and a reduction in complement C3/C4) have been reported (immune complexes and complement in non-IgE-mediated reactions).

In most cases patients are treated for the acute event in the casualty department and referral is made to an allergy specialist for further investigations and management. A detailed history is often helpful to elicit the potential cause of the reaction. In case of reactions where the suspected agent is known to provoke an IgE-mediated reaction, evaluation by SPT or radioallergosorbent testing (RAST) would be mandatory. For non-IgE-mediated reactions, diagnosis rests fully on a carefully obtained clinical history. In some cases of food-allergy or exercise-induced anaphylaxis, controlled challenges may be necessary to confirm

the diagnosis. In a minority of patients even after extensive investigation it may not be possible to elicit a cause, and such cases are termed 'idiopathic' anaphylaxis.

Management

Immediate

The mainstay in the management of an anaphylactic reaction is the provision of adequate oxygenation and circulatory support. Adrenaline (0.3–1 mg of 1:1000) should be administered immediately by IM injection. Most patients respond promptly to this dose if given early after the onset of the reaction. If blood pressure does not improve within 10 minutes, the dose should be repeated every 5–10 minutes until clear improvement occurs. If the clinical condition deteriorates rapidly, administration of adrenaline (1:10 000) by slow IV route under cardiac monitoring should be considered. In such cases plasma expanders (such as Dextran 70) and gelatin preparations may also be necessary to increase the intravascular volume and cardiac output. Monitoring central venous pressure or pulmonary capillary wedge pressure is helpful during intravascular volume replacement. When central venous pressure or pulmonary capillary wedge pressure is significantly

Table 5.1
The treatment of an anaphylactic reaction.

Specific measures
Lay the patient in a leg-raised position
Adrenaline: 0.5 mg IM. Repeat every 5–10 minutes if necessary. In case of a profound shock, adrenaline in a 1:10 000 solution is given as a slow 3–5 ml IV injection over 5 minutes or by continuous infusion using 1 ml of 1:1000 diluted in 500 ml of 5% dextrose infused at a rate of 0.25–2.5 ml/min
Chlorpheniramine maleate (Piriton): 10 mg slow IV/IM as a single dose
Hydrocortisone 100 mg IV/IM as a single dose

Supportive measures
Oxygen via mask 60–100%
Bronchodilator: Salbutamol 5 mg and ipratropium bromide 0.5 mg via nebulizer, 2–4 hourly
Resistant bronchospasm: Aminophylline as an infusion 0.5 mg/kg/hr
Monitor oxygen saturation if there is bronchospasm
Monitor BP every 5 minutes until patient is haemodynamically stable
T. prednisolone: Consider a short course, such as 20 mg stat. followed by 15 mg day 2, 10 mg day 3 and 5 mg day 4. This regimen is especially useful if an anaphylactic reaction occurs following administration of specific immunotherapy vaccine (depot preparations)
Severe refractory cases: noradrenaline 4 mg in 1 l of 5% dextrose at a rate of 2–12 µg/min (0.5–3 ml/min)
Patient on β blockers: 1 mg of glucagon in 1 l of 5% dextrose at a rate of 5–15 µg/min (5–15 ml/min)

Dosage of IM (1:1000; 1 mg/ml) adrenaline as per age:

Age	Volume (ml)
<1 year	0.05
1 year	0.1
2 years	0.2*
3–4 years	0.3*
5 years	0.4*
6–12 years	0.5*
Adult	0.5–1.0

(* suitable for robust children of this age; in case of underweight children, use half these doses) elevated, inotropic support with dopamine and dobutamine should be considered (*Table 5.1*).

Other measures include the administration of chlorpheniramine maleate (10 mg) and hydrocortisone (100 mg) by IM or IV routes. Chlorpheniramine is helpful because of its antihistaminic properties and hydrocortisone is given to suppress any late biphasic reaction from developing. Some physicians advocate the use of a short, rapidly tapering dose of prednisolone for additional benefit, especially if an anaphylactic reaction occurs following administration of a specific immunotherapy vaccine (depot preparations). Bronchospasm is often seen and, if this occurs, bronchodilators (such as salbutamol and ipratropium bromide) should be administered in a nebulized form together with 60–100% oxygen. Patients should be monitored continuously until improvement occurs and then be observed for at least 3–4 hours before discharge. Overnight observation may be necessary in some patients with severe reactions. Tracheostomy may be necessary in patients with severe upper airway obstruction due to laryngeal oedema.

A step-by-step management plan is summarized in *Table 5.1*.

Long term

The most important aspect in long-term management is patient education. If anaphylaxis is related to a specific allergen, then appropriate advice regarding allergen avoidance should be given. Other important measures include training the patient (and relatives and friends if necessary) in the use of an adrenaline auto-injector. It would be useful to provide the patient with a medi-alert badge clearly stating the patient carries an adrenaline auto-injector so as to alert paramedical staff in the event of an emergency.

Further reading

Ewan PW. Treatment of anaphylactic reactions. *Prescriber's J* (1997) **37**: 125–32.

Insect venom allergy

6

Introduction

Stinging insects are members of the Hymenoptera order (*Table 6.1*), which consists of apids, vespids and formicids. In the USA, allergic reactions to insect stings are reported by approximately 0.4% of the population. The number of deaths attributed to Hymenoptera stings is about 40 per year in the USA and between 2 and 9 deaths per year in the UK. In addition, some unexplained deaths (although attributed to heart failure) may in fact have been caused by stings.

All venom allergens are proteins and most are enzymes with molecular weights of between 13 000 and 50 000 daltons (*Table 6.2*). In addition to proteins and peptides, Hymenoptera venoms contain vasoactive amines, such as histamine, 5-hydroxytryptamine, acetylcholine, dopamine and norepinephrine.

Within the yellowjacket (*Vespula*) family there is strong cross-antigenicity and cross-allergenicity among venoms (see *Table 6.2*). There are rare individuals who react to

Table 6.1
The taxonomy of the Hymenoptera insect order.

Family	Subfamily	Scientific name	Common name
Apidae		*Apis mellifera*	Honeybee
		Bombus spp.	Bumblebee
		Megabombus spp.	
		Pyrobombus spp.	
		Halictus spp.	Sweatbee
		Dialictus spp.	
Vespidae	Vespinae	*Vespula* spp.	Wasp or yellowjacket
		Dolichovespula arenaria	Yellow hornet
		D. maculata	White-faced hornet
	Polistinae	*Polistes* spp.	Paper wasp
Formicidae		*Solenopsis invicta*	Fire ant
		S. richteri	
		Pogonomyrmex spp.	Harvester ant

Table 6.2
Selected biochemical and physicochemical properties of some Hymenoptera venom components.

Venom	Allergen	Common name
Honeybee	Api m 1	Phospholipase A_2
	Api m 2	Hyaluronidase
	Api m 3	Melittin
	Api m 4	Acid phosphatase
		Apamin
		Peptide 401
Vespids	Dol m 1	Phospholipase A_1
	Dol m 2	Hyaluronidase
	Dol m 3	Acid phosphatase
	Dol m 5	Antigen 5
		Kinin
		Mastoparan

one vespid species only but yellowjacket and paper-wasp extracts are commercially available that contain venoms from several species, so these individuals should not escape detection. There is little or no cross-reactivity between phospholipase A from the honeybee and vespid venoms, but hyaluronidases from the two different venoms may cross-react. This may explain the fact that some sting-sensitive individuals have positive skin test reactions to both honeybee and vespid venoms, but this might also be a result of sensitization to multiple venom components.

In Britain and the rest of Europe, wasps are a much more common cause of sting reactions than honeybees. Wasps or yellowjackets and honeybees are the most common cause of allergic sting reactions from the *Vespidae* and *Apidae*, respectively.

Clinical features (Table 6.3)

Acute hypotension and respiratory failure may occur after insect stings but most signs and symptoms resolve spontaneously or with therapy after

Table 6.3
The clinical features of bee and wasp sting reactions.

Immediate (within a few seconds or minutes)
Local reaction: erythema, swelling, pruritus

Generalized urticaria/angioedema
Laryngeal oedema
Bronchoconstriction
Hypotension; rarely myocardial infarction and arrhythmias complicating severe anaphylaxis

Delayed (6–8 hours)
Biphasic anaphylaxis
Fatigue
Immune complex glomerulonephritis, nephrotic syndrome
arthralgia

several hours. Immediate local reactions are normal and consist of transient pain and swelling at the sting site. Large local reactions are more extensive, often involving swelling and erythema of the whole limb that has been stung. Systemic reactions are generalized and involve signs or symptoms at a site remote from the sting. For example, a sting on the forehead resulting in angioedema of the eyelids would be classified as a local or large local reaction, whereas a sting on the foot that produced angioedema of the eyelids would be considered a systemic reaction.

Systemic reactions may involve generalized urticaria and pruritus, cutaneous or laryngeal oedema, broncospasm, abdominal cramping, nausea, and/or vomiting, and/or vascular collapse. These are IgE-mediated reactions that may be life-threatening if pulmonary or cardiovascular symptoms predominate. Persons who have experienced multiple previous episodes of anaphylaxis usually report stereotyped reactions, often with a perceived aura that appears shortly before the development of objective signs and symptoms. Toxic reactions are nonimmunological and occur after a person receives multiple stings within a short period of time or, rarely, one sting very close to a vein. The signs and symptoms are identical to those of systemic reactions, but in this case the symptoms are produced by exogenous vasoactive amines delivered in the insect venom, rather than endogenous vasoactive materials released as a consequence of venom allergen–IgE antibody interaction on mast cell surfaces. Intravascular haemolysis, adult respiratory distress syndrome, rhabdomyolysis, renal failure and disseminated intravascular coagulation may accompany fatal toxic reactions from Africanized honeybees.

Treatment

Local reactions to insect stings do not usually require any treatment but large local reactions are best treated with ice compression. For large uncomfortable local reactions, a three-day course of antihistamines may be beneficial. The general principles of the treatment of anaphylactic reactions to insect stings are similar to anaphylaxis of any cause (see Chapter 5 for details).

Patients whose signs and symptoms involve mainly cutaneous angioedema and urticaria (without hypotension or significant bronchospasm) can usually be discharged after the urticaria and bronchospasm have cleared. Biphasic anaphylactic episodes may occur. For the same reason, patients who initially experience significant broncospasm or hypotension (or who reside at some distance from medical care facilities) should either be admitted to hospital or be observed for 8–12 hours before discharge. In all cases of anaphylaxis, the patient should receive instructions on insect avoidance, a prescription for an epinephrine auto-injector and be referred to an allergist for further evaluation.

A carefully taken clinical history will usually permit identification of the culprit insect and accurate classification of the severity of the sting reaction. The worker honeybee stinger is barbed and, along with the attached venom sac, usually remains embedded in the sting victim. However, finding such an embedded sting apparatus is not absolute proof of a honeybee sting because vespid stingers and venom sacs also evulse in 4–8% of cases.

Honeybee venom is bacteriostatic and, therefore, honeybee sting wounds seldom become secondarily infected. Yellowjackets are predators and scavenge for food in rubbish bins and on dumps. Consequently, their stings frequently produce cellulitis. Yellowjackets are very aggressive and will sting without

provocation, particularly in late summer and autumn when their populations are highest and food supplies are dwindling.

Diagnosis

It is mandatory to investigate for the presence of specific IgE to bee and wasp venom in all patients with suspected insect sting allergy. Most centres prefer to evaluate this by measuring specific IgE levels in the peripheral blood. If this is significantly elevated there is no need to perform skin prick (SPT) or intradermal tests in view of the rare but real risk of provoking a systemic reaction. However, it is not unusual to encounter a minority of patients with a clinical history of insect sting allergy but who have a negative radioallergosorbent test (RAST). In such cases SPT or intradermal tests should be performed since SPTs are more sensitive than *in vitro* measurements.

Skin testing with insect venoms is the most rapid, sensitive and economic method to demonstrate venom-specific IgE antibodies. Intradermal tests are performed if the puncture test reactions are negative. Positive skin tests must be interpreted in relation to clinical history. The presence of a positive skin test denotes prior sensitization but does not predict whether a reaction will occur with the patient's next sting, nor does it discriminate between local and systemic reactions. Immunoassays are available commercially for *in vitro* measurement of venom-specific IgE antibodies. There is no correlation between the magnitude of the IgE antibody level and the degree of sensitivity of the patient, as assessed by deliberate insect sting challenges. The following clinical algorithm has been suggested to clarify the timing and significance of measuring IgE antibodies:

- Test patients as soon as referred.
- If the results are negative and the time elapsed since the sting is short, retest at 5–6 weeks.
- If the results are positive at 5–6 weeks and the history is suggestive of anaphylactic reaction, consider specific immunotherapy.
- If the results are negative at 5–6 weeks, no further testing is necessary.

The advantage of this algorithm is that approximately 80% of sensitive patients can be considered for immunotherapy immediately, thus reducing the risk inherent in not being treated while waiting to be tested. Measurement of venom-specific IgG antibodies has been suggested, but the data do not support the usefulness of this.

Desensitization treatment

Venom immunotherapy or desensitization should be considered in patients who have experienced a life-threatening systemic reaction to an insect sting and in whom an IgE-mediated reaction is demonstrable by SPT or RAST. Indications for venom immunotherapy are summarized in *Table 6.4*. The decision whether or not to administer venom immunotherapy is best made on an individual case basis and should take into account not only medical factors but also logistical, financial and other considerations unique to each patient and family. Specific immunotherapy in insect sting allergy is discussed in Chapter 10.

An algorithmic approach to the management of bee/wasp sting allergy is shown in *Figure 6.1*.

Conclusion

Collectively, the published data indicate that insect sting allergy is a self-limited process for many people: spontaneous remission of the sensitivity is greatest in children aged 16 years or under; and people at greatest risk of persistent sensitivity are those who have experienced more severe anaphylaxis,

Table 6.4
Indications for specific immunotherapy (SIT) in insect sting allergy.*

Grade of reaction	SIT
Anaphylaxis	Yes
Severe bronchoconstriction and/or laryngeal oedema	Yes
Generalized urticaria or/and laryngeal oedema without respiratory or cardiovascular involvement	? consider other risk factors, such as age, occupation, other medical problems (especially cardiovascular or respiratory system disorders)
Local reaction (small or large) only	No

* Specific immunotherapy should be administered only if there is evidence of an IgE-mediated reaction, i.e. a positive SPT or RAST together with clinical indications as summarized in this table.

regardless of their age or the number of intervening years since their previous sting reactions. Simple precautions may decrease the risk of insect stings (see Appendix I). People who have experienced generalized reactions to insect stings should be provided with epinephrine-containing kits for use in the event of a life-threatening reaction. These people should be advised to use the adrenaline auto-injector immediately when indicated and to seek medical attention at the nearest health centre.

For patients with severe systemic reactions to bee or wasp stings, immunotherapy is the only specific treatment currently available. Although venom immunotherapy significantly reduces the risk of future systemic reactions to the specific insect venom, there is still a very small but real risk of developing severe reactions, and all patients should be warned that they should still continue to carry their epinephrine auto-injector and not hesitate to use it if the need arises.

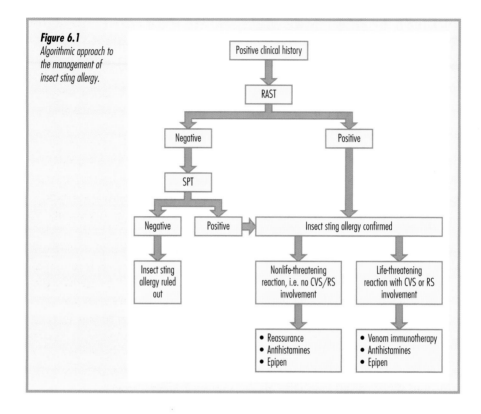

Figure 6.1
Algorithmic approach to the management of insect sting allergy.

Appendix I: Avoiding insect stings

- Avoid wearing shiny or brightly coloured clothing, flowery prints or black, as this seems to attract insects more than white, green, tan or khaki clothes.
- Wear shoes at all times when out of doors.

- Avoid using strong perfumes during the summer. Many products, such as suntan lotions, hairsprays, hair tonics and other cosmetics, contain strong perfumes.
- If possible, keep your arms and legs covered.
- Use an insect repellent containing diethyl-m-toluamide whenever you will

be outside for some time, especially if you have to be alone.

- If a bee or wasp comes near you, do not try to swat the insect but move away slowly and calmly. If the insect lands on you, try not to panic. Keep calm and be patient. The insect will usually fly away after a few seconds. Make sure you leave no crumbs or drink on your face, which will interest the insect.
- If you find many wasps or bees in your house or garden and suspect there may be a nest nearby – perhaps in the roof or in a nearby tree – phone the local authority or a pest control expert to come and remove the nest. Do not try to do this yourself.
- If you are planning to eat outside, find an area where there are no wasps or bees before you start eating. It is better to bring your picnic inside than to risk being stung.
- Food attracts insects. When outside, avoid open rubbish bins and keep food covered. Always look at what you are eating before you take a bite or sip a drink as wasps will slip into food and even into open drink cans. Boxed drinks with straws may be safer but keep an eye on the straw.
- Beekeepers should wear protective clothing when collecting swarms or honey.
- The bee leaves its stinger (with venom sac attached) in the victim. Because it takes a few minutes for all the venom to be injected, quick removal of the stinger is important. This is done with one quick scrape of the fingernail. The sac should not be picked up with thumb and forefinger because this squeezes in more venom.
- Always use your medication as instructed; it is better to inject yourself earlier, and perhaps unnecessarily, than later with serious consequences.

Source: Anaphylaxis Campaign information leaflet. Reproduced with permission.

Drug allergy

7

Introduction

Adverse drug reactions (ADR) constitute a common medical problem in all countries. It has been reported that allergic reactions to drugs account for 5–10% of ADRs and probability of allergic reaction for most drugs is 1–2%. Amongst many drugs involved in ADR, antibiotics and nonsteroidal anti-inflammatory drugs (NSAIDs) are at the top of the list. Although allergic reactions to drugs can affect individuals at any stage in their lives, it is seen most commonly in young or middle-aged adults. Epidemiological studies have shown that drug allergy is more frequently seen in women. Recent studies have linked HLA haplotypes to drug allergy: HLA-DQW2 in patients with aspirin-sensitive asthma, HLA-DRW2/DRW3 in patients with D-penicillamine allergy and HLA-B7DR2DR3 in patients with insulin allergy. A familial predisposition to antimicrobial allergy has also been reported. Children who have one parent allergic to an antimicrobial have a 15-fold higher risk of developing an allergic reaction to an antibiotic as opposed to a child whose parents are not allergic. Epidemiological studies have largely shown that, with a few exceptions, atopy *per se* does not constitute a risk factor for drug allergy. ADRs are more commonly seen in patients with HIV infection.

High molecular weight drugs such as antisera and insulin are more likely to produce allergic reactions than lower molecular weight drugs. The putative mechanisms underlying the development of allergic reactions are not completely understood. Consequently for most drugs there are currently no reliable tests to diagnose drug allergy. Several studies have shown involvement of both IgE and non-IgE-mediated mechanisms in drug allergy. The main non-IgE-mediated mechanisms include the activation of a complement pathway, direct mast cell degranulation, immune complex mediated-tissue insult, T-cell-driven and involvement of the kinin system.

The main emphasis of this chapter is on the clinical presentation of some of the most commonly encountered allergic reactions to drugs, their underlying mechanisms, diagnosis and management.

Special and common situations

Penicillin allergy

Amongst all drug allergies, allergic reactions to penicillin are the most common in general and hospital practice. This high prevalence (2%) is attributable to the extensive use of this class of drugs and their high protein avidity. Under physiological conditions, the β-lactam ring in the penicillin molecule opens and forms a covalent bond with serum proteins to form a 'penicilloyl or major determinant'. In patients with penicillin allergy more than 95% of specific IgE antibodies recognize this determinant. Covalent linkages with other portions of the molecule also occur and these are referred to as 'minor determinants' (penicilloate, penicilloyllamine, penilloate and benzylpenicilloyl-*n*-propylamine). Most anaphylactic reactions to penicillin have been shown to be mediated by the IgE specific to the minor determinant.

Diagnosis: Skin prick testing (SPT) is the gold standard in the diagnosis of penicillin allergy. In view of the formation of complexes with serum proteins, penicillin *per se* is an *inefficient* reagent for SPT. Penicilloyl-polylysine (PPL) is commercially available and has been shown to be sensitive and specific for the

IgE directed towards the major determinant. Similarly, minor determinant mixture (MDM) is also commercially available. Ideally, SPT should be performed at least 6 weeks after the patient has recovered fully from the allergic reaction, when other guidelines for the discontinuation of antihistamines apply (see Chapter 1). The negative predictive value of SPT to penicillin is now well established. In a patient with a positive clinical history and negative SPT, the probability of an allergic reaction to penicillin is 1% but anaphylaxis has never been reported in such patients. Studies have shown that 1–10% of patients with no previous history of penicillin allergy but with a positive skin prick test who receive this drug experience an allergic reaction. In addition, 50–70% of patients with a positive skin prick test and a history of a previous allergic reaction actually experience a further reaction upon re-exposure. Radioallergosorbent testing (RAST) for major and minor determinants is also available but is not as sensitive as SPT. SPT is contraindicated in patients with a history of drug-induced exfoliative dermatitis, Stevens-Johnson syndrome or Lyell's syndrome. In patients with proven allergy to penicillin and in whom treatment with penicillin is imperative (such as for neurosyphilis or bacterial endocarditis), acute penicillin

desensitization could be instituted. Several desensitization protocols have been described but these will not be discussed in this chapter. Desensitization is usually transient and requires continued exposure to the drug to maintain this state. Skin test and clinical reactivity return if penicillin is withdrawn for ≥ 48 hours. In view of cross-reactivities, most β-lactams and cephalosporins are contraindicated in patients with penicillin allergy. The only β-lactam that could be safely administered is the monolactam aztreonam because of its negligible cross-reactivity.

Aspirin and NSAID intolerance

It was in 1968 that Samter and Beers described the clinical syndrome of nasal polyposis, bronchial asthma and aspirin sensitivity. Since then a number of studies have looked into various aspects of this syndrome but the mechanisms underlying this drug allergy are still not fully understood. Aspirin and NSAIDs exert their anti-inflammatory effects by inhibition of the enzyme cyclo-oxygenase resulting in a shunt to the lipoxygenase pathway. Consistent with this view is an elevated baseline urinary leukotriene E4 and a further rise upon salicylate challenge. Allergic reactions to NSAIDs constitute the second most common cause of drug allergies seen in allergy clinics worldwide. Several studies have shown that approximately 10–30% of asthmatics are allergic to aspirin and NSAIDs and, interestingly, the underlying asthma is usually intrinsic. This class of drugs is known to exacerbate symptoms in 20–40% of patients with chronic idiopathic urticaria.

Several mechanisms, including IgE and non-IgE-mediated, have been proposed. These include T-cell-driven, neurohumoral acetylation, activation of an alternative complement pathway, the generation of leukotrienes and immune complexes. Thus, there is no single reliable test in diagnosis.

The usual clinical presentation of an acute reaction includes rhinoconjunctivitis, asthma, urticaria, angioedema, cutaneous rashes and anaphylactoid reactions. Delayed types of reactions are also common. Early reactions tend to occur between 30 minutes and 4 hours after ingestion and delayed reactions could occur up to 24 hours later.

More recently, a new syndrome of NSAID sensitivity and mite ingestion has been described by Blanco and co-workers. This syndrome is characterized by NSAID sensitivity and severe systemic reactions caused by ingestion of flour-based foods contaminated with *Dermatophagoides farinae* and mites of the *Acaridae* family. Patients have a previous history of respiratory hypersensitivity to dust mites.

The only way to confirm diagnosis is to undertake a double-blind placebo-controlled oral challenge test (OCT). An alternative approach would be to perform a bronchial challenge test (BCT) or a nasal challenge test (NCT) with lysine acetilic salicilate (LAS). NCT is much safer since LAS concentrations are 20 and 1000 times lower than BCT and OCT, respectively. More studies are required to validate these tests before they can be employed routinely in clinical practice.

The avoidance of aspirin and NSAIDs is a standard recommendation in patients with previous allergic reactions. Paracetamol, acetaminophen, sodium salicylate, choline salicylate, propoxyphane, salsalate, salicylamide and choline magnesium trisilicate do not cross-react and are useful alternatives. In patients with any underlying disease that warrants regular treatment with aspirin or any NSAIDs, desensitization can be initiated and maintained indefinitely as long as the patient is taking the regular daily treatment.

Muscle relaxants (Tables 7.1 and 7.2)

This class of drugs is most commonly implicated in anaphylactic/anaphylactoid reactions during general anaesthesia. The main mechanism underlying these reactions has been shown to be IgE-mediated mast cell degranulation and direct nonimmunological histamine-releasing ability from mast cells. The tertiary and quaternary ammonium groups of the molecule are the main allergenic determinants. Several *in vitro* studies have been carried out to study the histamine-releasing ability of these drugs and these are summarized in **Table 7.1**. These studies have clearly shown that muscle relaxants neither induce histamine from basophils nor induce *de novo* synthesis of vasoactive mediators in mast cells. However, it has been shown that these drugs can induce direct histamine release from mast cells obtained from different anatomical sites, and these responses show marked heterogeneity between different drugs, subjects and anatomical sites. This might explain the unpredictability of nonimmunological histamine release and the clinical manifestation of allergic reactions from a mild cutaneous type to severe hypotension. The sensitivity and negative predictive value of skin tests in the diagnosis of allergy to muscle relaxants have been shown to be excellent when performed by an allergy specialist. However, the poor positive predictive value of SPT to muscle relaxants invalidates their potential use as a screening test. Thresholds of positive reactions for SPT and intradermal test (IDT) for muscle relaxants are as follows: for atracurium and mivacuronium 1/10 and 1/100 dilutions are used for SPT and IDT respectively. For suxemethonium, gallamine, vecu-, ricu- and pancuronium neat extract and 1/10 dilution is used for SPT and IDT respectively. Kits for *in vitro* detection of a specific IgE by enzyme-linked immunosorbent assay (ELISA) are commercially available, but these are not as sensitive as SPT.

Opioids

Opioids have been shown to mediate anaphylactoid reactions by directly activating the mast cell, *albeit* a few IgE-mediated reactions have been reported. *In vitro* studies on morphine, buprenorphine and fentanyl have shown that none of these drugs is capable of inducing histamine release from basophils but that they show a marked heterogeneity in their effects on mast cells (see **Table 7.1**).

Table 7.1
In vitro *effects of muscle relaxants, opioids, benzo-diazepines, general anaesthetics and radiocontrast media on mast cells and basophils.*

Drug	De novo synthesis[*]	Basophil histamine release	Mast cell histamine release	
			Lung mast cell	Skin mast cell
Muscle relaxants				
Suxamethonium	nil	nil	nil	nil
d-tubocurarine	nil	nil	+ve	+ve
Vecuronium	nil	nil	+ve	+ve
Atracurium	nil	nil	+ve	+ve
Opioids				
Morphine	nil	nil	nil	+ve
Buprenorphine	+ve	nil	+ve	nil
Fentanyl	nil	nil	nil	nil
Benzodiazepines				
Diazepam	nil	nil	+ve	nil
Flunitrazepam	nil	nil	nil	nil
Midazolam	nil	+ve	+ve	nil
General anaesthetics				
Propofol	nil	nil	+ve	+ve
Ketamine	nil	nil	+ve	+ve
Thiopental	nil	nil	+ve	nil
Radiocontrast media	nil	+ve	+ve	+ve

[*]*Refers to mediators, including prostaglandin D_2 (PGD$_2$), platelet activation factors (PAF) and leukotriene C_4 (LTC$_4$), from human basophils and mast cells (in lung tissue, heart and skin). This is opposed to histamine and tryptase which are preformed mediators in mast cells.*

Table 7.2
The mechanisms underlying anaphylactic/anaphylactoid reactions to frequently implicated drugs and RCM.

Class	IgE-mediated	Non-IgE-mediated Complement driven	Direct activation
RCM	+/−	+	+
Opioids	+/−	−	+
GA (nonbarbiturates)	−	+	+
GA (barbiturates)	+	+	+
Muscle relaxants	+	−	+

Note: RCM: radio contrast media; GA: general anaesthetics.

Hypnotics and benzodiazepines

Whilst barbiturates are known to mediate their allergic reactions via specific IgE nonbarbiturate hypnotics such as propofol, althesin mediate their effects via non-IgE-mediated pathways (see *Table 7.1*). Although SPT and RAST are available for thiopentone, the negative predictive value is unknown. The *in vitro* effects of benzodiazepines on mast cells and basophils are summarized in *Table 7.1*.

Radiocontrast media (RCM)

Iodinated RCM are invaluable to radiologists in diagnostic procedures. Most of these compounds are derivatives of tri-iodinated benzoic acid, with an osmolality up to 3–5 times that of plasma. This hyperosmolality is at least in part responsible for some of the adverse reactions. Recently, agents with lower osmolality have been developed and this has significantly reduced the number of adverse reactions. The overall incidence of adverse reactions to RCM ranges between 4.6 and 8.5%, with a mortality of 0.002–0.009%.

RCM mediate their effects by the generation of anaphylatoxins, by the activation of a complement pathway and by inducing release of vasoactive mediators from mast cells and basophils from an unidentified pathway. The *in vitro* effects of RCM on mast cells and basophils are summarized in *Table 7.1*.

At present there are no tests available to diagnose allergy to RCM. In patients with a previous history of an allergic reaction to RCM of higher osmolality, a product with lower osmolarity is recommended. The prior administration of corticosteroids (32 mg methyl-prednisolone, 12 hours and 2 hours before procedure), together with H_1, H_2-receptor antagonists and ephedrine, has been shown to reduce the incidence of allergic reactions significantly. Desensitization has been attempted but this has not been shown to be superior to premedication with corticosteroids and antihistamines.

Local anaesthetics (LA)

Allergic reactions to LA are extremely rare. Most reactions are due to anxiety, vasovagal attacks, inadvertent intravenous injection, presence of epinephrine in the compound causing sympathetic stimulation and true allergic reactions attributable to preservatives such as bisulphites and parabens. Local anaesthetics can be immunochemically classified into 2 main groups:

(a) Benzoic acid esters: procaine, tetracaine, cocaine, benzocaine, butamben.
(b) Amide containing: lignocaine, mepivacaine, dibucaine, bupivacaine, etidocaine. Since there is no cross-reactivity between the 2 groups, amide LA free of preservative and epinephrine can be substituted for an ester and *vice versa* without allergy testing.

Skin prick and intradermal tests are not useful in diagnosis, and so an incremental drug challenge is used. This involves sequential intradermal injections (0.1–0.3 ml) starting at 1:10 000 dilution with progressive increments if no local/general reaction develops up to the concentration of the stock commercial solution. Subcutaneous challenge is performed starting at 0.1 ml of 1/10 000 and increasing the dose by 10-fold at 15 minute intervals. If well tolerated 0.5–1.0 ml of neat stock commercial solution can then be administered intramuscularly. If no reaction develops, true allergy to the local anaesthetic can be excluded.

Hypersensitivity reactions to drugs in HIV infection

Adverse reactions to drugs tend to occur more commonly in patients infected with HIV than in the general population. The most commonly described reaction is to trimethoprim-sulphamethoxazole (TMP/SMZ), which is used to treat *Pneumocytis carinii* pneumonia. This tends to manifest as a morbilliform pruritic rash during the first 7–10 days of treatment. More severe reactions, including, Stevens–Johnson syndrome, toxic epidermal necrolysis, hepatitis and interstitial pneumonias, have been described. Other drug reactions in this group of patients include reactions to penicillin, isoniazid, rifampicin, dapsone, sodium valproate, protease inhibitors and nucleoside reverse transcriptase inhibitors.

Adverse drug reactions are more common in patients with CD4 counts between 50 and 350 cells/mm^3. Although the precise mechanisms underlying these reactions are not well understood, recent studies have shown that the altered immunological status in HIV infection predisposes to these reactions rather than the chemical structure of the drugs *per se*. Depletion of intracellular glutathione in the lymphocytes, the induction cytochrome P450 by other drugs and the accumulation of toxic metabolites such as hydroxylamines have been implicated in adverse reactions.

Since most reactions are non-IgE-mediated, SPT and RAST are not helpful in diagnosis. The general approach recommended by most physicians is to desensitize patients directly without undertaking any formal challenge testing since most cases are clear cut. Challenges can be undertaken in less clear-cut cases.

Successful desensitization protocols have been reported with TMP/SMZ, anti-tuberculosis drugs and other drugs used for treating HIV infection.

A general approach to a case of drug allergy

The investigation and management of patients with a potential history of an allergic reaction to drugs are one of the most challenging tasks an allergologist encounters in his or her practice. The first and probably the most important step is to obtain a good clinical history and all the available information regarding the details of the drug(s) implicated in the allergic reaction, particularly dosage, route of administration, exact interval between administration of the drug and the onset of the reaction, and all clinical details regarding the reaction. It is extremely important to ascertain clinically whether or not it was a type I hypersensitivity reaction or was a type II, III or IV reaction.

As described previously, it is now evident that acute allergic reactions are mediated by several mechanisms and these could broadly be classified as:

- IgE-mediated
- non-IgE-mediated.

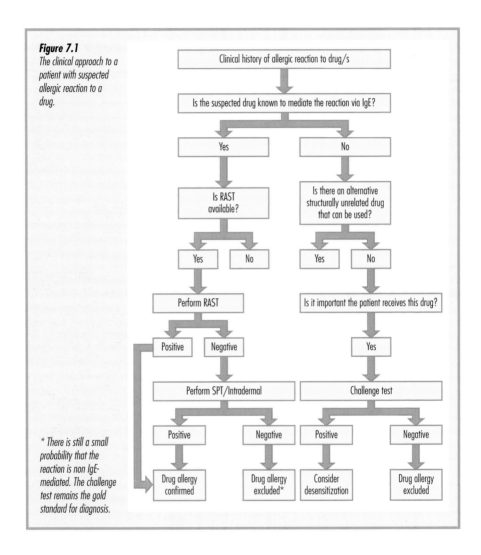

Figure 7.1
The clinical approach to a patient with suspected allergic reaction to a drug.

* There is still a small probability that the reaction is non IgE-mediated. The challenge test remains the gold standard for diagnosis.

For most drugs there is a paucity of information regarding the underlying mechanisms contributing to acute allergic reactions. Therefore, in cases where there is limited literature or where the drug is known to mediate allergic reactions by more than one pathway, screening for drug allergies by SPT, intradermal tests or RAST will not be sufficient to rule out drug allergy. In addition, for many drugs that are known to mediate an allergic reaction through a specific IgE, there are no data available regarding negative predictive values. Thus, 'challenge testing' remains the gold standard in the diagnosis of drug allergies. However, this method poses serious dangers in precipitating life-threatening allergic reactions. Consequently, the approach taken by most allergologists is to recommend treatment with an alternative drug that does not cross-react. In certain situations an alternative may not be available or is not as effective, in which case 'challenge tests' are carried out and, if positive, the patient should be considered for desensitization. *Figure 7.1* summarizes the clinical approach for use in a case of drug allergy.

Further reading

Anonymous. Mechanisms involved in immunological reactions to drugs. *Clin Exp Allergy* (1998) **28:** 3–91.

de Shazo RD, Kemp SF. Allergic reactions to drugs and biological agents. *JAMA* (1997) **278:** 1895–906.

Dykewics MS. Drug allergy. *Comprehensive Therapy* (1996) **22:** 353–9.

Genovese A, Stellato C, Marrella CV et al. Role of mast cells, basophils and their mediators in adverse reactions to general anaesthetics and radiocontrast media. *Int Arch Allergy Immunol* (1996) **110:** 13–22.

Poley GE Jr, Slater JE. Drug and vaccine allergy. *Pediatr Allergy Immunol Clin North Am* (1999) **19:** 409–22.

Food allergy

8

Introduction

Food allergy has been demonstrated to be a significant cause of life-threatening allergic reactions. The prevalence of food hypersensitivity is greatest in the first few years of life, affecting about 4–6% in the first year. Prospective studies from several countries indicate that about 2.5% of newborn infants experience hypersensitivity reactions to cows' milk in their first year of life. Up to 8% of children less than 3 years of age and approximately 2% of the adult population experience food-induced allergic disorders. Surveys from the UK indicate that 1.4–1.8% of adults experience adverse food reaction and that 0.01–0.23% of adults are affected by adverse reactions to food additives. Most children 'outgrow' (become tolerant of) their food hypersensitivity within a few years, except for foods such as peanuts and other nuts.

Food-induced allergic reactions are responsible for a variety of symptoms involving the skin, the gastrointestinal tract and the respiratory tract, and these can be caused by IgE-mediated and non-IgE-mediated mechanisms. About 35% of children with moderate-to-severe atopic dermatitis have skin symptoms provoked by food hypersensitivity, and about 6% of asthmatic children have a history of specific food-induced wheezing. However, many adverse reactions to foods (such as cows' milk) are seldom a result of true allergic reactions. In some cases, symptoms have been presumed to be allergic only because no other cause could be found and/or because the patient's symptoms improved when the food was withdrawn from the diet.

Food allergy can be broadly described under:

(a) *IgE-mediated reactions*
The presence of specific IgE (as established by skin prick testing (SPT) or radioallergosorbent testing (RAST)) and a reliable clinical history (i.e. a clear temporal relationship between ingestion of a food and onset of symptoms) constitute the two most important criteria in the diagnosis of food allergy.

(b) *Food intolerance or non-IgE-mediated reactions*
These are reproducible reactions to a specific food or food ingredient without any detectable specific IgE.

The precise underlying mechanisms leading to such reactions are not well understood.

Food allergens

Although hundreds of different foods are a part of the human diet, a relatively small number account for the vast majority of food-induced allergic reactions. In young children, milk, eggs, peanuts, soya bean and wheat account for approximately 90% of hypersensitivity reactions whereas, in adolescents and adults, peanuts, fish, shellfish and tree nuts account for approximately 85% of reactions. However, the increased accessibility of fresh fruits and vegetables from all over the world and our insatiable appetite for a more diversified and natural diet have resulted in an increase in allergic reactions to fruits (such as kiwi and papaya) and seeds (such as sesame, poppy and rape). The foods that have been found to cause IgE-mediated food allergy most commonly are listed in *Table 8.1*.

In some cases, the heating or cooking of foods may weaken or abolish allergenicity. Alternatively, in some cases, a food may only produce a reaction in its cooked form. Other foods have been found to become more troublesome after

Table 8.1
Common foods implicated in food allergy.

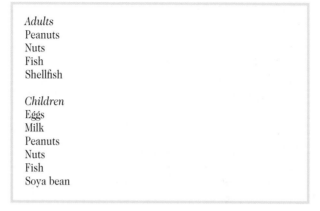

Adults
Peanuts
Nuts
Fish
Shellfish

Children
Eggs
Milk
Peanuts
Nuts
Fish
Soya bean

processing (e.g. the tinning of certain fish). The degree of ripeness of fruit may affect its allergenicity, as may the effect of storage. In general it appears that ripeness increases allergenicity and storage decreases it. In some cases there may be clear evidence that the allergic reaction relates simply to one variety of a food. This seems to be particularly noticeable in the case of potatoes and honey. However, a person may be allergic to several foods as a result of the presence of a specific IgE that can cross-react with certain immunoreactive epitopes that are present in several foods (*Table 8.2*).

Clinical features

Food allergy usually affects the skin, respiratory system, gastrointestinal tract and, in severe forms, the cardiovascular system (*Table 8.3*).

Gastrointestinal food hypersensitivity reactions

Since the gastrointestinal tract is the first system to confront food allergens, it is not surprising that a variety of gastrointestinal symptoms develop during an allergic reaction. These include nausea, vomiting, cramping pain, diarrhoea, abdominal distension and flatus.

Table 8.2
Cross-reactivity between food proteins and clinical cross-reactivity among members of plant and animal species.

Plant material	Cross-reacting foods	
Silver birch and hazel pollens	Parsnips Oranges Raw apples Onions Raw carrots	Tomatoes Raw potatoes Hazelnuts Raw celery
Grass pollen	Peaches Plums Apricots Cherries	
Mugwort pollen	Celery Apples Peanuts Kiwi fruit	
Ragweed pollen	Bananas Melon (watermelon, cantaloupe, honeydew)	
Latex	Bananas Chestnuts Avocados	Papayas Kiwi fruit Pineapples
Peanuts	Legumes (except lentils)	
Soya beans	Legumes	
Wheat	Other cereal grains	
Peanuts	Tree nuts	
Tree nuts	Other nuts	
Animal material	**Cross-reacting foods**	
Eggs	Chicken meat	
Cows' milk	Beef/veal	
Cows' milk	Goats' milk	
Beef/veal	Lamb	
Fish	Other fish species	

Table 8.3
The clinical manifestations of food hypersensitivity.

Type I, IgE-mediated	**Type II, antibody-dependent cytotoxicity**
Gastrointestinal reactions	? Milk-induced thrombocytopenia
Oral allergy syndrome (OAS)	
Infantile colic	**Type III, antigen–antibody complexes**
Nausea	? Coeliac disease
Vomiting	? Dermatitis herpetiformis
Diarrhoea	? Food-induced pulmonary hemosiderosis
Abdominal pain	? Cows' milk-induced intestinal blood loss
? Allergic eosinophilic gastroenteritis	? Arthritis
? Food-induced enterocolitis syndrome	
	Type IV, cell-mediated hypersensitivity
Cutaneous reactions	Coeliac disease
Urticaria and angioedema	? Food-induced enterocolitis syndrome
Atopic dermatitis	? Food-induced colitis syndrome
Contact dermatitis	? Food-induced malabsorption syndrome
	? Dermatitis herpetiformis
Respiratory reactions	? Food-induced pulmonary haemosiderosis
Rhinoconjunctivitis	Mechanism(s) unknown
Asthma	Migraine headache
Laryngeal oedema	Occult gastrointestinal blood loss
Generalized reactions	
Anaphylactic shock	

Symptoms typically develop within minutes to 2 hours of consuming the responsible food allergen and consist of nausea, abdominal pain, colic, vomiting and/or diarrhoea. These can be accompanied with symptoms such as urticaria, angioedema, breathlessness/wheeze and, in severe forms, hypotension leading to collapse.

Oral allergy syndrome

This syndrome is seen in patients who are sensitized to pollen (tree pollens in particular). It results from a cross-reactivity of antibodies against the heat-labile protein 'profilin' that is present in pollen and certain fresh fruits and vegetables. This protein is denatured by heating/cooking. Hence patients develop symptoms only when they eat fresh fruits/vegetables but not when these foods are cooked. The symptoms are confined to the oropharynx and include pruritus, tingling and swelling of the lips, tongue and pharynx, but they are almost never life-threatening. Almost all symptoms occur within 30 minutes and they are generally short lived.

It is estimated that about 40% of patients suffering from hay fever from various pollens (especially birch, ragweed and mugwort) develop symptoms upon eating fresh fruits and vegetables. Patients allergic to ragweed may experience oral allergy syndrome (OAS) after contact with various fresh melons (e.g. water melons, cantaloupes and honeydews) and bananas. Symptoms may be more prominent after the ragweed season, corresponding to the seasonal rise in ragweed-specific IgE levels. Patients allergic to birch pollen may have symptoms after the ingestion of raw potatoes, carrots, celery, apples, hazelnuts and kiwi.

SPT with the commercial extracts of fruits are often reliable and the currently recommended technique is the prick-to-prick, which involves pricking the fresh fruit with a lancet or needle and then pricking the patient's skin. The use of antihistamines may ameliorate oral symptoms but caution must be exercised, and the diagnosis must be made certain so as not to mask early symptoms of a systemic reaction. Successful birch pollen immunotherapy has been shown to alleviate oral symptoms in a small number of patients.

Cutaneous food hypersensitivity reactions

The skin probably represents the second most frequent target organ in food hypersensitivity reactions (*Table 8.3*). Ingestion of food allergens may provoke the rapid onset of cutaneous symptoms or aggravate more chronic conditions. Acute urticaria and angioedema are believed to be among the most common symptoms of food-induced allergic reactions. Since the onset of symptoms follows within minutes of ingestion of the responsible allergen, the cause-and-effect nature of the reaction is generally obvious to the patient. Symptoms are caused by the activation of IgE-bearing mast cells in circulating food allergens, which are absorbed and circulate rapidly throughout the body.

Food allergy seldom accounts for chronic urticaria and angioedema. In large-scale studies, food allergy was implicated in only 1.4% of adults with chronic urticaria. In another study it was reported that 31%

of the children had positive skin tests to food but that only 4% had symptoms confirmed by double-blind placebo-controlled food challenges (DBPCFC). Food additives (both dyes and preservatives) are also frequently implicated in chronic urticaria but rarely confirmed by appropriate challenges.

There is now substantial evidence to link food allergy with eczema. In selected patients, an elimination diet has resulted in a significant improvement of the eczema.

Food-induced generalized anaphylaxis

Generalized anaphylactic reactions have long been recognized as a complication of food allergy. Reports indicate that food allergy is the single most common cause of anaphylaxis as seen in hospital emergency departments. Food-induced anaphylaxis accounts for about one third of cases, twice as many as provoked by Hymenoptera stings. It is estimated that there are about 100 fatal cases of food-induced anaphylaxis in the USA each year. The foods most frequently associated with severe reactions in the western world are peanuts, tree nuts, seafood, eggs and milk.

The time of onset of the reaction after food ingestion is variable, but symptoms are typically noted within a few minutes. Initial symptoms are likely to be swelling or itching of the lips, tongue or throat, nausea and vomiting. In some patients, the initial symptoms are rapid loss of consciousness and cyanosis. In some cases of fatal food-induced anaphylaxis, children initially had mild symptoms and were thought to be improving only to have severe symptoms up to $2\frac{1}{2}$ hours later. Patients may develop cardiovascular symptoms, including hypotension, vascular collapse and cardiac dysrhythmias, in addition to cutaneous, respiratory and gastrointestinal symptoms.

Food-dependent exercise-induced anaphylaxis

Food-dependent exercise-induced anaphylaxis is a rare and unusual form of anaphylaxis that occurs only when the patient exercises within 2–4 hours after ingesting a specific food. The incidence of food-dependent exercise-induced anaphylaxis appears to be increasing, possibly because of the increased popularity of exercising in the past decade. Anaphylaxis may occur when a patient exercises within 2–4 hours after ingesting a food, but in the absence of exercise the patient can ingest the food without any apparent reaction as long as the incriminated food (or foods) has not been ingested within the past several hours. Patients with specific food-dependent exercise-induced anaphylaxis generally have asthma and other atopic disorders. SPT is positive to the food that provoked the symptoms and, occasionally, there is a history of reaction to the food when the patient was younger.

This disorder appears to be twice as common in females as in males and is most prevalent in patients in their late teens to late thirties. Interestingly, the menstrual cycle sometimes influences the development of symptoms in food-dependent exercise-induced anaphylaxis in women, with the symptoms reported being most pronounced just before menstruation. The exact mechanism or mechanisms involved in this disorder are unknown and several foods have been implicated, including wheat, shellfish, fruit, milk, celery and fish. The specific management of this disorder involves identifying the food or foods that cause the reaction and avoiding them before any anticipated exercise. As with other food-allergic patients, these patients must have injectable epinephrine and a *per os* antihistamine available at all times.

Allergic eosinophilic gastroenteritis

As the name suggests, this disorder is characterized by eosinophilic infiltration of the gastrointestinal tract, stomach and small intestine in particular, and most patients have multiple food allergies. Symptoms depend on the organ involved and the extent of eosinophilia. Stomach involvement can present as reflux, abdominal pain, vomiting and, in children, failure to thrive and refusal of food. Intestinal involvement can present as malabsorption, diarrhoea, obstruction and, rarely, ascites.

Diagnosis is based on clinical history and demonstration of eosinophilic influx in the gastrointestinal tract (on mucosal biopsies). Eosinophilia disappears/ subsides and this is paralleled by clinical improvement when the patient is maintained on an elemental diet for 6–8 weeks. In cases of multiple sensitivities demonstrated in SPTs, a period of strict elimination followed by careful reintroduction of foods, one after the other can help establish foods that are to be avoided. In some cases foods cannot be implicated, and there are reports that the disorder has been treated successfully with oral sodium cromoglycate, or prednisolone.

Diagnosis

Given increasing public awareness of food allergy and the frequent misperception that various symptoms are caused by food-induced allergic reactions, the physician must retain some scepticism throughout the evaluation and rely on objective measures to arrive at the final diagnosis. Overdiagnosis of food allergy has led to malnutrition, eating disorders and psychosocial problems (as well as family disruption), whereas underdiagnosis leaves the patient suffering unnecessarily and may result in both growth failure and permanent physical impairment.

The diagnostic approach to suspected adverse food reactions begins with a careful medical history and physical examination. The goal of this exercise is to determine whether the patient is likely to have experienced an adverse reaction to food and whether there is an underlying IgE-mediated mechanism.

Table 8.4 lists a number of alternatives that should be considered in differential diagnosis.

If there is an obvious food provoking the reaction, the following facts should be ascertained:

- The quantity of food ingested.
- The length of time between ingestion and the development of symptoms.
- Whether ingesting the suspected food produced similar symptoms on other occasions.
- Whether other factors (e.g. exercise or alcohol ingestion) are necessary to induce the symptoms.
- The length of time since the last reaction to the food occurred.

Table 8.5 lists some of the principles that should be kept in mind when assessing the patient's history.

In chronic disorders provoked by food allergies (e.g. atopic dermatitis, asthma and allergic eosinophilic gastroenteritis), medical history has poor predictive accuracy. In routine allergy practice, several patients with symptoms of chronic fatigue syndrome or fibromyalgia are referred to rule out underlying food allergies as a cause: in most cases there is no demonstrable allergy.

Physical examination

During physical examination, attention should be directed towards the cutaneous, gastrointestinal and respiratory systems and towards detecting the presence of

Table 8.4
Differential diagnosis of adverse food reactions.

Gastroinestinal disorders

Structural abnormalities
Hiatus hernia
Pyloric stenosis
Tracheoesophageal fistula
Hirschsprung's disease

Enzyme deficiencies (primary Vs secondary)
Disaccharidase deficiency (lactase, sucrose–isomaltase, glucose–galactose)
Galactosaemia
Phenylketonuria

Malignancy

Other
Pancreatic insufficiency (cystic fibrosis, Schwachman–Diamond syndrome)
Gall bladder disease
Peptic ulcer disease

Contaminants and additives

Flavourings and preservatives
Sodium metabisulfite
Monosodium glutamate
Nitrites/nitrates

Dyes
Tartrazine
? Other azo dyes

Toxins
Bacteria (*Clostridium botulinum,*
  Staphylococcus aureus)
Fungal (aflatoxin, trichothecene, ergot)
Seafood-associated disorders
Scrombroid poisoning (tuna, mackerel)
Ciguatera poisoning (grouper, snapper, barracuda)
Saxitoxin (shellfish)

Infectious organisms
Bacteria (*Salmonella, Shigella, Escherichia coli, Yersinia, Campylobacter*)
Parasites (*Giardia, Trichinella, Anisakis simplex*)
Virus (hepatitis, rotavirus, enterovirus)
? Mould antigens

Accidental contaminants
Heavy metals (mercury, copper)
Pesticides
Antibiotics (penicillin)

Pharmacological agents
Caffeine (coffee, soft drinks)
Theobromine (chocolate, tea)
Histamine (fish, sauerkraut)
Tryptamine (tomato, plum)
Serotonin (banana, tomato)
Tyramine (cheeses, pickled herring)
Glycosidal alkaloid solanine (potatoes)
Alcohol

Psychological reactions

Table 8.5
Some principles for use in the assessment of patients with food allergies.

- Patient's history is notoriously inaccurate.
- Food allergy is most common in young children, especially with atopic dermatitis.
- Relatively few foods are responsible for the vast majority of allergic reactions.
- It is rare for patients to react to more than three foods.
- When a child with food allergy has 'new' or 'multiple' food allergies, it is most likely that he or she is ingesting 'hidden' sources of common food allergens.
- Except in gastrointestinal allergies, most food-induced allergic symptoms develop within minutes to a few hours of ingesting the food allergen.
- True food allergies generally involve 'classical' signs and symptoms affecting the skin, gastrointestinal and/or respiratory systems.
- Subjective or behavioural symptoms as a sole manifestation of food allergy are very rare.
- 'Adverse reactions' to dyes and additives are rare.

atopic features, which are more commonly found in patients experiencing IgE-mediated reactions. The general nutritional status of the patient and any physical signs of underlying nonallergic disorders should be noted. Patients experiencing severe atopic dermatitis or asthma should prompt a more aggressive evaluation.

Diet diary cards

Diet diary cards are frequently used as an adjunct to medical history. Patients are instructed to keep a chronologic record of all foods ingested over a specified period of time, including items just placed in the mouth (such as chewing gum). Any symptoms experienced by the patient are also recorded. The diary is then reviewed to determine whether there are any obvious associations between the foods ingested and the symptoms experienced. As opposed to the medical history, this approach gathers information on a prospective basis and is not so dependent on a patient's memory. Nevertheless, interpretation of diary cards may be extremely cumbersome and difficult and should be used in highly selected cases where clinical history is not obvious but where there is a high index of suspicion.

Elimination diets

Elimination diets are used in both the diagnosis and management of adverse food reactions. Once certain foods are suspected of provoking allergic disorders, they are completely omitted from the diet. The success of these diets depends on the identification of the correct allergen or allergens, the patient's ability to maintain a diet completely free of all forms of the offending allergen and the assumption that other factors do not provoke similar symptoms during the period of study.

Unfortunately, this is rarely accomplished. If symptoms resolve while a patient is maintaining an elimination diet, some form of food challenge is generally required to confirm the diagnosis of food allergy, especially in chronic disorders such as atopic dermatitis or asthma. With gastrointestinal allergies, endoscopy and biopsy (showing significant resolution of gut pathology after 6–8 weeks on an elimination diet) will confirm that the implicated food or foods were most likely responsible for the disorder.

Laboratory studies

During the history and physical examination, the physician should establish whether the patient's findings implicate a food-induced allergic disorder and whether an IgE-mediated or non-IgE-mediated mechanism is most likely responsible. SPT and RAST may be useful in delineating the specific foods responsible for IgE-mediated disorders, whereas laboratory studies are of limited value in non-IgE-mediated disorders.

A practical approach to diagnosing food allergy

The diagnosis of food allergy remains a clinical exercise dependent on a careful history, selective skin tests or RAST (if an IgE-mediated disorder is suspected), an appropriate exclusion diet and blinded provocation. Currently there is no evidence of any diagnostic value for food-specific IgG or IgG_4 antibody levels, food antigen–antibody complexes, lymphocyte activation or sublingual or intracutaneous provocation. In gastrointestinal disorders where prechallenge and postchallenge biopsy studies are required for diagnosis, blinded challenge may not be necessary.

An exclusion diet eliminating all foods suspected by history or skin testing (for IgE-mediated disorders) should be conducted for 1 or 2 weeks in suspected IgE-mediated disorders and food-induced enterocolitis and colitis. Diets may need to be extended for up to 12 weeks in other gastrointestinal disorders (such as allergic eosinophilic gastroenteritis) after appropriate biopsies. If the patient does not improve, it is unlikely that food allergy is involved. However, in cases of atopic dermatitis and chronic asthma, other precipitating factors may make it difficult to discriminate the effects of the food allergen from other provocative factors.

A diagnostic approach in a case of suspected food allergy is illustrated in *Figure 8.1*.

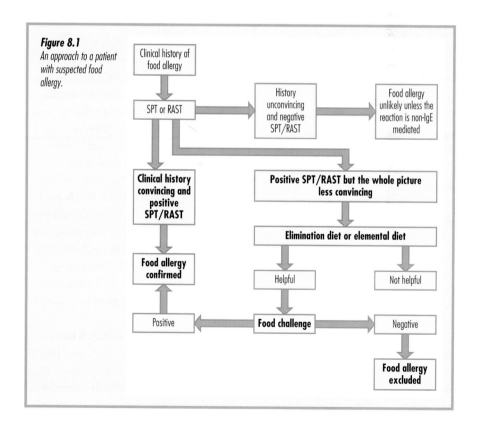

Figure 8.1
An approach to a patient with suspected food allergy.

Therapy

Once the diagnosis of food hypersensitivity is established, the only proven therapy is strict elimination of the offending allergen. Prescribing therapeutic elimination diets should be undertaken with the same consideration as given to prescribing medications – both may result in unwanted side-effects. Elimination diets may lead to malnutrition and/or eating disorders, especially if they include a large number of foods and/or are used for extended periods of time. Patients and their families must be taught to study food labels to detect potential sources of hidden food allergens. The elimination of a single food can be very difficult. For example, milk may be designated on the food label in several ways (such as casein, caseinate, whey, lactalbumin, nougat, natural flavouring, caramel flavouring and hydrolysed protein). In addition, milk protein is typically found in 'nondairy' creamers and soya bean cheeses, in lunchmeats and hot dogs and, not uncommonly, in soya bean or rice frozen desserts.

Various 'high-risk' situations must be avoided, such as eating at buffets, receptions, some restaurants, friends' homes, school cafeterias and ice-cream shops. In certain situations, airborne food particles may induce allergic reactions (which are occasionally fatal) in highly sensitive patients (e.g. patients allergic to fish or shellfish in seafood restaurants, patients allergic to eggs standing next to cooking scrambled eggs and patients allergic to peanuts in aeroplanes where passengers are opening peanut packs). Certain foods may contain aspirin or yeast, and patients with a history of allergy to these should avoid specific items (see Appendices I and II). The complexity of the therapeutic elimination diet for the patient increases with each additional food allergy, leading to increased frustration or lack of compliance (or both).

Clinical reactivity to food allergens is generally very specific and patients rarely react to more than one member of a botanical family or animal species. Consequently, therapeutic elimination diets should not be based on the exclusion of food families but be based on individual foods proven to induce allergic symptoms. In patients in whom multiple food allergies have been identified, it is imperative to enlist the services of a dietitian who is knowledgeable in dealing with food exclusion diets and has experience of patients allergic to foods.

Patients with oral allergy syndrome can generally consume cooked or processed forms of the implicated food or vegetable.

Thus a person with oral allergy syndrome to apples can eat apple sauce and apple pie and can drink pasteurized apple juice. Alternatively, classic food allergens (such as milk, eggs, peanuts, soya bean, wheat and tree nuts) involve proteins that are very resistant to processing and heat, and these can trigger a reaction in a sensitive individual in even minute quantities in any form. The risks and difficulties faced by food allergy patients at home, at school, in restaurants and while grocery shopping will have a tremendous impact on patients' lives. A safe motto to follow is: 'If you cannot read the label, do not eat the food!' Patients with very sensitive peanut or tree nut allergies should not eat desserts away from home or have peanuts or tree nuts in their homes.

Weeks or months of exclusion of the reactive food may lead to the possibility of reintroduction without a reaction. This is known as *tolerance* and its maintenance depends on establishing the threshold of both frequency and quantity for that person.

Intolerance of additives in foods and medicines

Preservatives are added to many commercially produced foods to prevent the deterioration of food, and they are important in the prevention of food poisoning caused by bacterial contamination. They are also essential to modern ways of processing, packaging and transporting grocery goods. Fresh foods without preservative (sugar and salt act as preservatives) have to be eaten within a limited period to avoid the risk of microbial contamination. Alternative ways of prolonging storage times include canning, freezing, freeze-drying and bottling.

Antioxidants prevent the degradation of fats and fat-soluble vitamins. A wide number of flavourings and flavour enhancers is now added to foods. Other food additives include emulsifiers, stabilizers and a wide range of sweeteners and thickeners.

Whilst it is possible for any food additive to cause problems in a sensitive individual, it appears that some can cause more problems than others. A summary of the most widely investigated additives and the problems they cause is given in *Table 8.6*.

Medications (such as H_1 and H_2-antihistamines, ketotifen, cromones, corticosteroids and leukotriene inhibitors) have been used in an attempt to modify the symptoms of food-induced allergic disorders. Antihistamines may partially

Table 8.6
Food additives that can cause problems.

Additive	Source	Possible effects
Antioxidant preservatives E320 and E321	Used to preserve oils and fats. Widely found in commercially prepared packaged foods which contain fats and oils	Have been shown to trigger both asthma and urticaria in susceptible subjects
Nitrate and nitrite preservatives E249–E251	Used to preserve and stabilize the colour of some cooked meats (for example ham and bacon) and cheeses	Have been shown to trigger both urticaria and headache in susceptible subjects
Benzoate preservatives E210–E218	Preservatives used in fruit squashes, fruit syrups, fizzy drinks and some medicines. Benzoates occur naturally in some foods, particularly honey and cranberries	Have been shown to trigger urticaria, and possibly asthma and eczema. May cause behavioural effects in some hyperactive children
Sulphite preservatives E220–E228	Sulphites occur naturally in the fermentation of yeast. Some are therefore always present in wines and beers. Sulphites may be added to beers, wines and fruit juices. They are often used in preparing dried fruits (some have very high levels), seafood, gelatin, dehydrated vegetables, pickles, preserved meats, sausages, fruit salads and green salads. Sulphites may be sprayed on to prepared foods to preserve them (for example, in salad bars and restaurants)	Susceptible asthmatics may react to sulphite when a sulphite-containing food is eaten. Very susceptible asthmatics may even react when sulphur dioxide fumes are released from fruit juice or wine to which sulphite has been added. Sulphite sensitivity has also been shown to be a cause of rhinitis and urticaria. Sulphite sensitivity can be very difficult to suspect and detect
Glutamate flavour enhancers E620–E625	Certain foods contain significant amounts of glutamate naturally. These include Parmesan cheese, meat extracts, vegetables or tomato concentrates, peas and mushrooms. Monosodium glutamate is widely used as a flavouring and is popular in oriental cooking	Glutamates have been shown to provoke asthma in a few susceptible asthmatics. However, the proportion affected is not certain. Urticaria may rarely be provoked. In some sensitive individuals, a characteristic reaction (the Chinese restaurant syndrome) occurs, which includes a tingling skin, headache, nausea, sweats, palpitations and even fainting

mask symptoms of oral allergy syndrome and IgE-mediated skin symptoms, but overall they have minimal efficacy. Oral corticosteroids are generally effective in treating chronic IgE-mediated disorders (e.g. atopic dermatitis or asthma) or non-IgE-mediated gastrointestinal disorders (e.g. allergic eosinophilic oesophagitis or gastroenteritis and dietary-induced enteropathy), but the steroid side-effects are generally unacceptable.

The protective effect afforded by the oral administration of sodium cromoglycate (Nalcrom, RPR) can be utilized in the management of food allergic conditions in two ways:

1 To cover planned breaks in an elimination diet either for single meals or over a period of a few days. The dose required to reduce the effects of a single challenge should be determined in advance and will usually be in the range of 50–150 mg for infants, 100–200 mg for children and 400–600 mg for adults. If more than one dose is given during 24 hours the total daily dose should not exceed 40 mg/kg. The drug should not be used if there is any history of anaphylactic reactions to foods. In cases of food allergy this use of oral sodium cromoglycate should be exceptional rather than routine, and an elimination diet remains the treatment of first choice.

2 In conjunction with an elimination diet when the diet alone does not provide adequate control of the symptoms.

Given the difficulty of avoiding food allergens, it must be assumed that patients will experience accidental ingestion. Approximately 35–50% of patients allergic to peanuts will experience an accidental peanut ingestion within a 3 to 4-year period. If they are at risk of severe anaphylaxis (i.e. they have experienced a previous severe reaction or have asthma), they must be given an auto-injectable epinephrine and antihistamine injection and a written emergency plan describing their allergy, potential symptoms, medications to be given and emergency telephone numbers to call. It must be stressed to all the people involved that treatment must be initiated without delay in high-risk patients and that they must be taken to an emergency facility for further evaluation and treatment. About one third of patients with systemic anaphylaxis will experience a biphasic response.

Immunotherapy has been tried for the treatment of food-induced allergic disorders. Using 'standard' immunotherapy in patients who have experienced peanut-induced anaphylaxis, it was demonstrated that a minority of patients could tolerate larger quantities of peanuts for a prolonged period after rush therapy, but the adverse reaction rate was unacceptable for standard clinical practice. Consequently, alternative strategies for the treatment of patients with food allergy are being explored.

Conclusion

About 2% of the population is affected by various food-induced allergic disorders. A number of well characterized food-induced allergic disorders have been delineated. Patients afflicted by these disorders may be accurately diagnosed through systematic evaluation (including medical history, physical examination, SPT, specific-IgE *in vitro* testing, diet diaries, elimination diets and oral challenges). Once the appropriate diagnosis has been made, patients must be educated to avoid the specific food allergen or allergens and to treat allergic reactions in case of an accidental ingestion. It is hoped that new diagnostic tests, better food labelling laws and better awareness in the medical community and the general public will lead to more accurate food allergy diagnoses, fewer incidences of accidental food ingestion and decreased food-related fatalities.

Appendix I: A salicylate-free diet

Salicylates (found in aspirin) also occur naturally in some foods. It is important that, whilst following this diet, patients avoid all aspirin and aspirin-containing medicines.

Foods with a high salicylate content (more than 2 mg/100 gr food)

Fruit	Fresh pineapple, prunes, blackcurrants, raspberries, dates, sultanas, currants, raisins, fresh apricots, tinned cherries, oranges
Vegetables	Gherkins
Nuts	Almonds, water chestnuts
Miscellaneous	Tomato ketchup, liquorice, honey, curry powder, oregano, paprika, rosemary, thyme

Foods with a medium salicylate content (between 1–2 mg/100 g food)

Fruit	Strawberries, gooseberries, fresh cherries, blackberries, tinned apricots, melon, tinned pineapples
Vegetables	Peppers, radishes, endive, courgettes, tinned mushrooms, olives, tomato purée
Nuts	Peanuts
Miscellaneous	Mints, liqueurs, port, rum

Foods with a low salicylate content (less than 1 mg/100 g food)

Fruit	Plums, rhubarb, apples, figs, grapefruits, pears, grapes, peaches, kiwi fruits, watermelons, nectarines, avocado pears
Vegetables	Parsnips, spinach, okra, onions, broad beans, aubergines, french beans, marrow, cucumbers, broccoli, carrots, cauliflowers, beetroots, sweetcorn, tomatoes, tomato juice, turnips, watercress
Nuts	All except those on above lists
Miscellaneous	Jam, marmalade, ice cream, Worcestershire sauce, vinegar and other sauces containing vinegar, tomato soup, beer, cider, sherry, brandy, wine

Foods with no salicylate content

Fruit	Bananas, Golden Delicious apples, tinned pears
Vegetables	Peeled potatoes, swede, Brussels sprouts, peas, leeks, lettuce, cabbage, celery, bean sprouts, lentils, black-eyed beans, soya beans
Cereals	Barley, buckwheat, maize, oats, rye, rice, wheat
Miscellaneous	Meat, fish, milk, eggs, cheese, sugar, syrup, gin, vodka, whisky

Appendix II: A low yeast diet

AVOID FOODS CONTAINING YEAST

All breads containing yeast

FOODS ALLOWED

Soda or sourdough breads, crispbreads, rice cakes, etc. (check labels, particularly crispbreads)

Buns, teacakes, rolls, crumpets, hot-dogs, breadcrumb toppings (e.g. fish cakes)

In moderation – plain scones, pastries, plain cakes (no dried fruit), fruit tarts

Sausages, meatloaves and beefburgers and other meat products that contain bread

Any plain meat, fish or pastry

Alcoholic drinks, beer, wine, spirits, cider

Non-alcoholic beverages and fruit juices

Yeast extracts, including Marmite, Bovril, stock cubes and some soups and gravy granules (always read the labels carefully)

Fray Bentos stock cubes. Soups free from yeast extract. Simple gravy browning

Vinegar and pickled foods, ketchup, mayonnaise, salad cream, soy sauce

Salt, pepper, herbs, spices, lemon juice

Coleslaw, vegetable or potato salad, mushrooms

All other fresh vegetables, salads and potatoes

Vitamin tablets containing B vitamins

Yeast-free vitamins

Further reading

Burks AW. Childhood food allergy. Pediatric allergy and immunology. *Immunol Allergy Clin North Am* (1999) **19**: 397–407.

Bush RK, Taylor SL. Clinical and diagnostic approaches to adverse reactions to food and drug additives. Middleton E, Reed CE et al., eds. *Allergy: Principles and Practice* (5th edn) (Mosby-Year Book, Inc., St Louis, MO, 1998).

Daniels MA. Oral diagnostic challenges. Comprehensive care in the allergy/asthma office. *Immunol Allergy Clin North Am* (1999) **19**: 75–82.

Edwards AM. Oral sodium cromoglycate: its use in the management of food allergy. *Clin Exp Allergy* (1995) **25 (suppl 1)**: 31–33.

Food allergy and intolerance. Report of a BSACI Special Interest Group, June 1992–September 1993. *Clin Exp Allergy* (1995) **25 (suppl 1)**: 1–44.

Food allergy: current knowledge and future directions. *Immunol Allergy Clin North Am* (1999) **19**: (small book).

Gern JE, Lemanske RF. Pediatric allergy: can it be prevented? Pediatric allergy and immunology. *Immunol Allergy Clin North Am* (1999) **19**: 233–52.

Hourihane JO'B. Peanut allergy – current status and future challenges. Review. *Clin Exp Allergy* (1997) **27**: 1240–46.

Metcalfe DD. Food allergy. Allergy and immunology. *Primary Care; Clinics in Office Practice* (1998) **25**: 819–29.

Ortolani C. Food allergy. *Allergy* (1995) **50 (suppl 20)**: 5–81.

Plaut M. New directions in food allergy research. Workshop synopsis. *J Allergy Clin Immunol* (1997) **100**: 7–10.

Sampson HA. Food allergy. Part 1. Immunopathogenesis and clinical disorders. Food allergy. Part 2. Diagnosis and management: current reviews of allergy and clinical immunology. *J Allergy Clin Immunol* (1999) **103**: 981–9.

Simon RA. Differential diagnosis of allergic disease: masqueraders of allergy. Adverse reactions to food and drug additives. *Immunol Allergy Clin North Am* (1996) **16**: 137–76.

Steinman HA. 'Hidden' allergens in foods. Rostrum. *J Allergy Clin Immunol* (1996) **98**: 241–50.

Atopic dermatitis (eczema)

9 Definition

Atopic dermatitis (AD) is synonymous with atopic eczema and usually begins in childhood (infantile eczema). AD is a chronically relapsing, pruritic, exanthematous dermatosis of uncertain aetiology that is characterized primarily by an allergic diathesis as well as erythema, oozing, crusting, excoriations, lichenification and dehydration of the involved skin surfaces. It has a characteristic distribution on the face and extensor surfaces in infants, but tends to affect the flexures in children and adults. More than 50% of sufferers have a personal or family history of asthma or hay fever.

Incidence

About 30% of the population is atopic. Recent reports of AD suggest an overall cumulative prevalence of 0.5–1.5% by 7 years of age and 2–10% in adults. There has been a two to threefold increase in cases over the last 30 years suggesting that environmental factors, such as the progressive urbanization of society and increasing levels of irritants and pollutants in homes, may be affecting disease expression. Certain populations who migrate from areas of low disease prevalence (such as Africa or Asia) to areas of high prevalence (such as Europe or New Zealand) have experienced an increased incidence of AD. Overall, males and females are affected with equal incidence and severity, and clear racial and ethnic predilections have not been established. Seasonal variation does play a role in the prevalence, with exacerbations occurring primarily in the winter.

Natural history

Hospital-based studies show that 75% of patients develop their dermatitis before 6 months of age and 80–90% by 5 years of age. Fewer than 2% of patients develop the disease after 20 years of age. AD improves with age: about 50% of patients are clear of their dermatitis by 13 years of age. However, remission at puberty with recurrence in late adolescence or in the early twenties is not uncommon. Few cases persist beyond the age of 30 years. Furthermore, over 50% of patients with AD develop asthma and approximately 75% develop allergic rhinitis as they outgrow AD. However, patients with AD can have nonallergic as well as allergic triggers similar to patients with asthma and allergic rhinitis.

Clinical features

The diagnosis of AD is made on clinical criteria. Diagnostic criteria for AD have been based primarily on the presence or absence of clinical features of the disease (*Table 9.1*). In children, the diagnosis of AD requires the presence of at least three out of four major, and at least three minor, criteria. A UK working party recently developed a minimum set of diagnostic criteria validated for adult, paediatric and non-Caucasian ethnic groups with atopic dermatitis for use in hospitals and the community, and these are shown in *Table 9.2*.

Intense pruritus and cutaneous reactivity associated with a lowered 'itch threshold' are hallmarks of AD. Several skin lesions are also commonly seen. In patients with chronic AD, all three skin reaction patterns may coexist in the same individual. AD may start at any age but the peak age of onset is 2–6 months. The disease affects both sexes and may persist, with periodic exacerbations and remissions, into adulthood. Itching often

Table 9.1
Diagnostic criteria for atopic eczema

Major criteria: at least three of the following:

1 Pruritus
2 Personal or family history of atopy (asthma, allergic rhinitis, atopic dermatitis)
3 Chronic or chronically relapsing dermatitis
4 Typical morphology and distribution (face and extensors in early childhood and flexures with lichenification in adolescence)

Minor criteria: at least three of the following:

1 Xerosis
2 Hand/foot dermatitis
3 Cheilitis
4 Elevated serum IgE
5 Immediate (type 1) skin test reactivity
6 Facial pallor/facial erythema
7 Perifollicular accentuation
8 Tendency to skin infections (i.e. *Staphylococcus aureus* and herpes simplex)
9 Icthyosis, keratosis pilaris or hyperlinear palms
10 Early age of onset
11 Anterior neck folds
12 Recurrent conjunctivitis
13 Anterior subcapsular cataracts
14 Keratoconus
15 Pityriasis alba
16 Course influenced by emotional factors
17 Food intolerance
18 Pruritus with sweating
19 Intolerance of wool
20 Orbital darkening
21 Nipple eczema
22 Dennie–Morgan folds/lower eyelids
23 White dermographism

Table 9.2
UK diagnostic criteria for atopic dermatitis.

The diagnosis of atopic dermatitis requires that the patient has:

- An itchy skin condition (or parental report of scratching or rubbing in a child) plus three or more of the following:
- Onset below 2 years of age (not used if child is under 4 years).
- History of skin crease involvement (including cheeks in children under 10 years).
- History of a generally dry skin.
- Personal history of other atopic disease (or history of any atopic disease in a first-degree relative in children under 4 years).
- Visible flexural dermatitis of cheeks/forehead and outer limbs in children under 4 years).

Source: Williams HC, Burney PGJ, Pembroke AC et al. *Br J Dermatol* (1994) **131:** 406–16. Reproduced with permission.

---

disturbs sleep and leads to extensive excoriation. Sites predisposed to rash change with growth and development. The appearance of the disease varies with age and is classically described in three phases.

Infantile phase

The rash starts characteristically on the cheeks but may affect any part of the skin. Generally, the nappy area is spared. Extensor involvement of the limbs may develop when the child begins to crawl. Initial lesions are oedematous, erythematous papules, which may become confluent. They are often markedly excoriated with exudation and crusting. When the dermatitis flares, intermittent morbilliform erythema may appear on the trunk. Affected infants are typically fussy from sleep deprivation because of pruritus and often are uncomfortable, fretful and may not eat well. Secondary infection and lymphadenopathy often occur. More than 50% of babies gradually develop the flexural pattern of the childhood phase, though some are clear of the dermatitis by 18–24 months.

Childhood phase

The exudative oedematous lesions reduce in frequency and severity and lichenification becomes predominant. Thickened excoriated skin, with increased skin markings, affects the antecubital and popliteal fessae, and the sides of the neck, wrists and ankles. Exudative lesions may occur on the hands and discoid patches of eczema are occasionally present on the limbs. In Afro-Caribbean, Asian and Chinese children, persistence of an extensor pattern with marked lichenification may be seen. Older children who have severe atopic eczema are frequently asthenic and may have difficulties at school.

Adult phase

The lichenification involvement of the flexures and hands is similar to the childhood phase. Pigmentary changes to the neck are common. In more severely affected patients flushing and itchy erythema of the face on a background of lichenification occur. This can spread to the upper chest, back and arms.

Figures 9.1 and *9.2* illustrate dermatological manifestation of atopic dermatitis.

Differential diagnosis

In most patients the diagnosis of AD is straightforward. However, scabies should always be excluded (*Table 9.3*). Scabies can present as a pruritic skin disease. However, distribution in the genital and axillary areas, the presence of linear lesions and the results of skin scrapings may help distinguish it from AD. It is especially important to recognize that an adult who has eczematous dermatitis with no history of childhood eczema and without other atopic features may have contact dermatitis but, more importantly, cutaneous T-cell lymphoma needs to be ruled out. Ideally, biopsies should be sent from three separate sites because histology may reveal spongiosis and cellular infiltrates similar to AD. In addition, eczematous rash suggestive of AD has been reported with HIV. A contactant should be considered in patients whose AD does not respond to appropriate therapy. Typical distribution for suspected contactant may be suggestive. However, allergic contact dermatitis complicating AD may appear as an acute flare of the underlying disease rather than the more typical vesiculobullous eruption. Proper diagnosis depends on confirmation of a suspected allergen with patch testing.

Figure 9.1
A young adult with atopic dermatitis affecting his forearm and arm.

Source: Courtesy of Professor P Friedman, Department of Dermatology, University of Southampton.

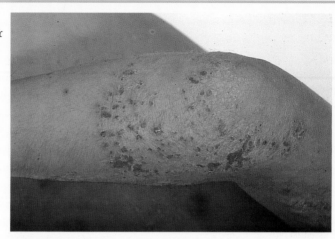

Figure 9.2
A young adult with flexural atopic dermatitis of lower limbs.

Source: Courtesy of Professor P Friedman, Department of Dermatology, University of Southampton.

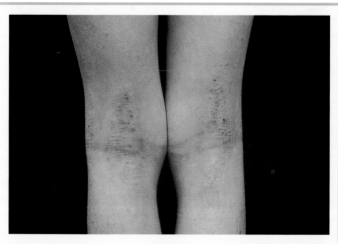

Table 9.3
Differential diagnosis of atopic dermatitis.

Immunodeficiencies
Wiskott–Aldrich syndrome
DiGeorge syndrome
Hyper-IgE syndrome
Severe combined immune deficiency
Histiocytosis X
Ataxia-Telangiectasia

Metabolic diseases
Phenylketonuria
Tyrosinaemia
Histidinaemia
Multiple carboxylase deficiency
Essential fatty acid deficiency
Pyridoxine (vitamin B6) and niacin
 deficiency
Zinc deficiency

Neoplastic disease
Cutaneous T-cell lymphoma
Histiocytosis X
Sézary syndrome
Netherton's syndrome

Infection and infestation
Candida
Herpes simplex
Staphylococcus aureus
Scabies
Fungal infections
Pityriasis rosea
Erysipelas

Dermatitis
Contact (allergic or irritant)
Seborrheic
Ichthyosis
Varicosis dermatitis/stasis eczema
Nummular eczema
Chronic dermatosis
Psoriasis

Drug reactions
Photodermatitis
Acrodermatitis enteropathica
Graft-versus-host diseases

Comparison of the features of seborrhoeic and atopic dermatitis

	Seborrhoeic dermatitis	*Atopic dermatitis*
Age of onset	Less than 2 months	2–6 months
Pruritus	Uncommon	Common
Distribution of rash	Napkin area, axillae, scalp	Face, forearms, shins
Family history of atopy	30% of patients	Greater than 50%
IgE levels and RAST to eggs and milk	Normal IgE, negative RASTs	Elevated IgE, positive RASTs
Prognosis	Good; clears by 6 months May progress to atopic dermatitis	Chronic and relapsing associated with asthma and hay fever

Source: Disease management of atopic dermatitis: a practice parameter. *Ann Allergy Asthma Immunol* (1997) **79**: 197–211. Reproduced with permission.

Immunodeficiency states (e.g. Wiskott–Aldrich syndrome, infections, thrombocytopenia) should be considered in infants whose disease is unusually severe or when there is recurrent infection, failure to thrive, malabsorption or petechiae. Flexural eczema may arise from the secondary dissemination of a contact allergy, such as nickel dermatitis. Many patients with occupational dermatitis, hand dermatitis, pompholyx, discoid eczema or asteototic eczema are atopic.

Complications

Quality of life

AD has a profoundly detrimental effect on the lives of patients and their families. Nocturnal scratching commonly has a destructive effect on sleep patterns and, in severe cases in childhood, this can lead to behavioural problems and can interfere with the functioning of the family.

Cutaneous infection

Staphylococcus aureus almost always colonizes inflamed atopic skin and may cause flares of AD as a result of activation of the immune system. In these cases, antibiotic treatment may help control the dermatitis even in the absence of frank infection. Obvious staphylococcal infections (e.g. impetigo) are more common in atopic patients. Occasionally, infected atopic skin can be complicated by the presence of β-haemolytic streptococcal infection.

Patients with AD have an increased susceptibility to infection or colonization with a variety of other organisms. These include viral infections with herpes simplex virus, molluscum contagiosum and infections with human Papillomavirus. Superimposed dermatophytosis may cause AD to flare. Patients with AD appear to have a threefold increase of *Trichophyton rubrum* infections compared with controls. *Pityrosporum ovale* has also been associated with a predominantly head and neck distribution of AD.

Ocular problems

Ocular complications associated with AD can lead to significant morbidity. Atopic keratoconjunctivitis is always bilateral and symptoms include itching, burning, tearing and copious mucoid discharge. It is frequently associated with eyelid dermatitis and chronic blepharitis and may result in visual impairment from corneal scarring. Vernal conjunctivitis is a severe bilateral, recurrent chronic inflammatory process of the upper palpebral conjunctiva usually occurring in younger patients. It has a marked seasonal incidence, often in the spring. The associated intense pruritus is exacerbated by exposure to irritants, light or by sweating. Examination of the eye reveals papillary hypertrophy or 'cobblestoning' of the upper inner eyelid surface. Keratoconus is a conical deformity of the cornea believed to result from persistent rubbing of the eyes in patients with AD and allergic rhinitis. Anterior subcapsular cataracts may develop during adolescence or early adult life.

Patients with severe AD may develop bilateral cataracts. Peak incidence is at 15–25 years of age. They are also at risk of developing corticosteroid-induced cataracts.

Viral infections

Patients with AD may develop generalized herpes simplex infection or eczema herpeticum. Parents should be told about this serious complication and warned that, if they have an active cold sore, they should not kiss or cuddle children with AD. Eczema herpeticum must be suspected in infected areas that have tiny erosions or crusts, and IV acyclovir therapy considered.

In the past, atopic children were advised not to be vaccinated against smallpox because of the risk of dissemination of vaccinia. However, other routine vaccinations are safe.

Growth retardation

About 10% of children with severe AD are small for their age. Whether this results from their disease or from topical corticosteroid therapy is debatable. The evidence suggests that dermatitis is the cause because intensive therapy can promote a growth spurt. Whatever the cause, children with severe disease should have their height and weight monitored.

Investigations

There is little need for investigation of the average patient with AD. IgE levels, skin prick tests (SPTs) and radioallergosorbent tests (RASTs) are usually unhelpful for management and merely confirm the atopic nature of the individual. The appropriate investigations should be performed only if an immunodeficiency underlying the dermatitis is suspected. Elevated serum eosinophilic cationic protein or depressed cord blood-derived polyunsaturated fatty acid levels in high-risk infants may have some utility as markers for AD. Complications such as antibiotic-resistant staphylococcal infection, β-haemolytic streptococci or herpes simplex should be detected by the appropriate swabs for culture. Patch testing may be considered if the skin condition deteriorates and may help identify any sensitivity that has developed to topical preparations (e.g. lanolin and, more recently, hydrocortisone).

Management

Management of AD is influenced by many factors, including age, the extent of the disease, the sites of involvement and home circumstances. AD is a chronic, relapsing condition and must be treated accordingly.

Education

Education of the patient and parents of a child with AD is crucial and should be supported with written information. They must understand the condition and the expectations of therapy. Treatment can greatly improve the disease, but no therapy can completely prevent relapse. Medical management should provide satisfactory control of the condition and minimize the unwanted side-effects of therapy.

Trigger factors

It is helpful to explain to patients that underlying their condition is an overly sensitive skin, and that inflammation can be triggered by a combination of factors. Environmental factors, including contact irritants and allergens, climate, sweating, aeroallergens, microbial organisms, certain foods and stress, all have been shown to trigger AD in susceptible individuals (*Table 9.4*). Indeed, recent studies in patients sensitive to house dust mite have shown that active implementation of allergen avoidance measures results in significant improvement of eczema.

Treatment

First-line therapy

Among the primary objectives in the successful management of acute AD are rehydration of the stratum corneum, anti-inflammatory treatment, interruption of the itch–scratch cycle and eradication of micro-organisms. Other important considerations are allergy testing and the removal of precipitating factors.

Emollients
Rehydration is achieved by daily baths in warm water (at least one per day) in

Table 9.4
Some precipitating factors in atopic dermatitis.

- Contact irritants and allergens (mechanical irritation, soaps, solvents, preservatives, detergents, wool).
- Climate (especially winter and low humidity).
- Diaphoresis.
- Aeroallergens, including the house dust mite (*Dermatophagoides pteronyssinus*), moulds, pollen and animal dander.
- Microbial organisms (*Staphylococcus aureus*, *Pitysporum* yeasts, *Candida* organisms and *Trichophyton*).
- Foods (eggs, milk, soya bean, nuts, fish, shellfish and wheat).
- Stress/psyche.

which a small amount of an oil and a mild emulsification agent are added. A small amount of mineral oil whisked in water is a low-cost alternative. The purpose of the oil is to help replace the effect of natural cutaneous lipophilic barriers that seal hydration within the skin. Many practitioners advocate the addition of a small amount of baking soda to bathwater for pruritus, but this benefit should be weighed against the drying potential of baking soda.

Hydrophobic creams that have good dispersion properties in water may be used in place of soap when bathing younger children. These creams have excellent cleansing properties and low potential for irritancy. If soap is preferred, a mild nonscented type may be used. Baby shampoo or a suitably mild shampoo may be used to manage scalp dermatitis.

After bathing, the skin should be patted dry to avoid mechanical irritation. A suitable topical moisturizing agent (either medicated or nonmedicated) should be applied to the skin within approximately 3 minutes to seal in moisture. Some of the best bland emollients are hydrophobic/ointment-based and include petrolatum. These preparations can be very greasy. These more elegant products are less occlusive and, therefore, less effective as moisturizers. They should be recommended if compliance with the greasier products becomes an issue. Frequent application of moisturizers throughout the day helps to maintain a high level of hydration in the stratum corneum.

Topical anti-inflammatory agents (corticosteroids)

Topical anti-inflammatory agents (corticosteroids) are the cornerstone of treatment for acute flares. The role of corticosteroids should be explained to the patient and parents. The strength of the corticosteroid required varies (*Table 9.5*). For mild cases of AD, a suitable low-potency (class VI or VII) steroid should be applied at least twice daily to help decrease inflammation and further build the integrity of the skin. If applied immediately after bathing in place of a bland emollient, the steroid preparation acts as a medicated moisturizing agent. Treatment should commence with hydrocortisone 1.0% cream mixed with an equal amount of hydrocortisone ointment 1.0%, which combines the moisturizing aspects and potency of an ointment with the elegance of a cream. Generally, topical corticosteroids should be applied using the weakest effective strength until the inflammation settles. The treatment should be repeated when the eczema returns.

The strength and efficacy of commercially available corticosteroids depend on the vehicle of formulation as well as the chemical structure. In general, ointment preparations have much more powerful anti-inflammatory properties than their cream counterparts. Steroid ointments are more occlusive and greasy than creams and help the skin to retain moisture, but they are messy to use and may increase sweat retention and pruritus in warmer climates. Creams are well tolerated but less effective as moisture retention agents than ointments. Gels and lotions, which have alcohol or water bases, are well tolerated on hairy areas such as the scalp, but they also are drying agents and may sting areas of compromised integument. For this reason, they are generally not recommended in the treatment of AD. Topical corticosteroid and tar mixtures applied to lichenified skin can be soothing and help to reduce the strength of the corticosteroid required. Antiseptics (e.g. clioquinol) or antibiotics (e.g. hydrocortisone acetate 1% and fucidic acid (Fucidin, Leo)) could be added to the corticosteroid preparation to reduce staphylococcal contamination.

Occasionally, usually in adults, deterioration in the patient's dermatitis may be caused by the development of a contact allergy to one of the topical preparations. Patch testing may then be considered to identify the cause.

Table 9.5
Topical glucocorticoid potency ranking.

Group I
Betamethasone dipropionate 0.05% (cream & ointment)
Clobetasol propionate 0.05% (cream & ointment)
Diflorasone diacetate 0.05% (ointment)
Halobetasol propionate 0.05% (cream & ointment)

Group II
Amcinonide 0.1% (ointment)
Betamethasone dipropionate 0.05% (cream & ointment)
Desoxymethasone 0.25% (cream)
Desoxymethasone 0.05% (gel)
Diflorasone diacetate 0.05% (ointment)
Fluocinonide 0.05% (cream, gel, ointment & solution)
Halcinonide 0.1% (cream)
Mometasone furoate 0.1% (ointment)

Group III
Amcinonide 0.1% (cream & lotion)
Betamethasone dipropionate 0.05% (cream)
Betamethasone valerate 0.1% (ointment)
Desoxymethasone 0.05% (cream)
Diflorasone diacetate 0.05% (cream)
Fluocinonide 0.05% (cream)
Halcinonide 0.1% (ointment & solution)
Triamcinolone acetonide 0.1% (ointment)

Group IV
Hydrocortisone valerate 0.2% (ointment)
Flurandrenolide 0.05% (ointment)
Fluocinolone acetonide 0.025% (ointment)
Mometasone furoate 0.1% (cream)

Group V
Betamethasone dipropionate 0.05% (lotion)
Betamethasone valerate 0.1% (cream)
Fluticasone acetonide 0.025% (cream)
Fluticasone propionate 0.05% (cream)
Flurandrenolide 0.05% (cream)
Hydrocortisone valerate 0.2% (cream)
Prednicarbate 0.1% (cream)

Group VI
Alclometasone dipropionate 0.05% (cream & ointment)
Betamethasone valerate 0.05% (lotion)
Desonide 0.05% (cream)
Flucinolone acetonide 0.01% (cream & solution)
Triamcinolone acetonide 0.1% (cream)

Group VII
Hydrocortisone hydrochloride 1% (cream & ointment)
Hydrocortisone hydrochloride 2.5% (cream, lotion & ointment)
Hydrocortisone acetate 1% (cream & ointment)
Hydrocortisone acetate 2.5% (cream, lotion & ointment)
Pramoxine hydrochloride 1.0% (cream, lotion & ointment)
Pramoxine hydrochloride 2.5% (cream, lotion & ointment)

Source: Disease management of atopic dermatitis: a practice parameter. *Ann Allergy Asthma Immunol* (1997) **79**: 197–211. Reproduced with permission.

Antihistamines

Itching is the major symptom of AD and no therapy specifically combats it. Nocturnal itching can be soothed by sedative antihistamines. Antihistamines can also be given for severe flares during the daytime if the patient is resting at home or in hospital. Nonsedating antihistamines have a minimal effect.

Second-line therapy

Most cases of AD can be relieved by constant attention to the details described above. Patients who do not improve should be reviewed to check for compliance, to exclude antibiotic resistance and to consider second-line treatment.

Topical corticosteroids

For more severe cases of AD, topical steroids of mild to high potency (classes III–V) may be applied for brief periods of no longer than 1–2 weeks. Class VII steroids should not be applied to the face or skin fold regions of the body. Localized areas of lichenification and excoriation on the limbs can be improved by nocturnal bandaging with zinc oxide or tar-impregnated cotton bandages.

Antibiotics

Secondary infection is present in most cases of flaring atopic eczema and frequently exacerbates disease. *Staphylococcus aureus* is the most common causative organism, necessitating appropriate anti-staphylococcal therapy. Widespread infection should be treated with oral antibiotics and the selection of an antimicrobial should be guided by the incidence of *S. aureus* resistance and allergy. Cephalexin, dicloxacillin, erythromycin and amoxycillin-clavulanate are reasonable choices. For more localized infection, topical antimicrobials such as mupirocin, bacitracin, 3% precipitated sulphur in petrolatum or 3% iodochlorohydroxyquin in 1% hydrocortisone may be applied to affected areas twice daily. Simultaneous intranasal application of mupirocin twice daily for 10 days helps eliminate staphylococcal carrier status. If *Pityrosporum ovale* fungal infection is suspected (a common yeast present in the head and neck region and diagnosable by 5% potassium hydroxide preparation), a suitable antifungal topical preparation, such as ketaconazole cream or shampoo, should be added to the treatment regimen. Bacterial and fungal cultures and sensitivities should be obtained if there is any question about the identity of an infecting organism or microbial resistance. In severe cases, hospital admission for intensive topical treatment will settle the flare and allow the dermatitis to be controlled better at home.

Allergen management

Allergy testing to foods may be useful in identifying possible precipitants of AD attacks in very young children. For accurate skin testing, antihistamines must be discontinued one week and topical steroids two weeks prior to testing. Skin testing is carried out best during periods of relative remission. Avoiding substances believed to precipitate attacks is helpful, although hyposensitization injections have not been efficacious.

Other factors in the treatment of AD should be considered. Known contact allergens and irritants, including preservatives, perfumes, antiseptics, soaps, solvents and wool clothing, should be eliminated from the child's environment. The effect of climate and low humidity could be minimized. Family stressors in older children can be addressed with the aid of family counselling. Treatment failures should be examined closely for the possibility of resistant organisms, contact dermatitis to a medication (e.g. preservatives in steroid preparations, bacitracin) or for parental noncompliance.

Third-line therapy

Immunomodulators such as azathioprine, cyclophosphamide, thalidomide, cyclosporine and tacrolimus are effective in severe adult atopic eczema. In children, cyclosporine has been used with caution for the treatment of extremely recalcitrant AD. Tacrolimus, a topical immunomodulator that has an encouraging safety profile, has been studied in paediatric populations and may soon be approved for the treatment of paediatric AD. Natural and artificial ultraviolet light have been shown to alleviate symptoms (presumably as a result of effects on the immune system) and may have some benefit in the treatment of AD in older children. However, their usefulness is limited by the availability of UV lighting systems, cost and patient compliance.

Several forms of alternative therapy, including Chinese herbal teas, hypnotherapy, fatty acid supplementation, elimination of cows' milk or highly restrictive diets (in the absence of known food allergy), have been advocated and have been shown to be efficacious in the treatment of AD in some trials. Chinese herbal teas contain up to 10 different herbs, many of which have anti-inflammatory, antihistaminic and immunosuppressant activity. Omega-6 fatty acids presumably increase prostaglandins E (PGEs) and thymic hormone activity, resulting in suppression of IgE production and stimulation of T_{H1} cells. Further research is needed to explore the full potential of these interventions.

Prognosis

In most cases, the prognosis is good for children who have AD. Most cases of atopic eczema resolve by adulthood, although 20–40% of atopic children remain atopic as adults. Frequent follow-up is important early in the disease course to assess responsiveness to treatment and parental compliance with treatment regimens for younger children. Bath oil soaks with daily applications of moisturizers and the avoidance of precipitating factors should be continued during the maintenance period. Antibiotics and steroids should be reserved for disease flares, and antihistamines may be used on an as-needed basis. Good treatment habits developed early in life will provide the framework for long-term successful disease control.

Further reading

Boguniewicz M, Leung DYM, Atopic dermatitis. In: Middleton E, Reed CE et al., eds. *Allergy: Principles and Practice* (5th edn) (Mosby-Year Book, Inc., St Louis, MO, 1998).

Burks W, James JM. Atopic dermatitis and food hypersensitivity reactions. *J Pediatr* (1998) **132:** 132–6.

David TJ. Atopic eczema. *Prescriber's J* (1995) **35:** 199–205.

Disease management of atopic dermatitis: a practice parameter. *Ann Allergy Asthma Immunol* (1997) **79:** 197–211.

Holden CA. Dermatology: atopic dermatitis. *Medicine* (1997) **25:** 37–41.

Kennedy MS. Comprehensive care in the allergy/asthma office: evaluation of chronic eczema and urticaria and angioedema. *Immunol Allergy Clin North Am* (1999) **19:** 19–33.

Knoell KA, Greer KE. Atopic dermatitis. *Pediatr Rev* (1999) **20:** 46–52.

Sampson HA. Pathogenesis of eczema. *Clin Exp Allergy* (1990) **20:** 459–67.

Sampson HA, Sicherer SH. Food allergy: current knowledge and future directions. Eczema and food hypersensitivity. *Immunol Allergy Clin North Am* (1999) **19:** 495–517.

Shaw JC. Differential diagnosis of allergic disease: masqueraders of allergy. Allergic and nonallergic eczematous dermatitis. *Immunol Allergy Clin North Am* (1996) **16:** 119–35.

Immunotherapy

10

Introduction

Immunotherapy began in the early 1900s and was first applied to allergic rhinitis. In 1911, Noon prepared pollen extracts based on the weight of the pollen and he administered these extracts subcutaneously at 1–2 week intervals. He observed that patients receiving injections of grass pollen extract had diminished ocular allergen challenge reactions. The response to the administration of these allergens was dose dependent, but large doses of allergen extracts could provoke a systemic reaction.

Immunotherapy antigens have now expanded to include trees, weeds, animal dander, house dust mites and stinging insects. Over the last decades, controlled studies have been undertaken to define the role of allergen immunotherapy in the treatment of allergic rhinitis, allergic conjunctivitis, insect anaphylaxis and asthma. It is only useful for allergic disease and has no role in the management of various types of nonatopic manifestations. Indiscriminate and inappropriate use of immunotherapy for nonallergic symptoms has contributed to the erroneous view held by some practitioners that it is generally an ineffective form of treatment.

The immunologic basis of immunotherapy

Allergen immunotherapy is the administration of increasing quantities of allergens to patients with IgE-mediated allergic rhinitis, asthma or stinging insect anaphylaxis. Immunotherapy moderates an abnormal immune response and has multiple immunologic effects:

- A rise in specific IgG (speculated to have a blocking effect against the antigen administered).
- A 'switch' of the immune response from the T_{H2} to T_{H1} profile (results in down regulation of IL-4 and upregulation of γ-interferon).
- A long-term decrease in specific IgE against the antigen.
- A reduction of mediators released in allergic response (by mast cells and basophils).
- A decrease of serum eosinophil chemotactic activity and histamine-releasing factors.
- A reduction of the cellular inflammation associated with specific allergen challenge.

Medical effectiveness

Venom sensitivity

Immunotherapy continues to be the treatment of choice for the prophylaxis of insect sting allergy. The availability of purified venoms and subsequent commercial distribution provided a major breakthrough in the treatment of insect-allergic individuals. Initial studies documented the almost 100% effectiveness of venom immunotherapy in preventing resting anaphylaxis. The goal of venom immunotherapy is to provide protection from subsequent stings in individuals considered to be at risk as defined by a history of insect sting anaphylaxis and the presence of venom-specific IgE (positive skin test). Venoms are available for honeybees, yellowjackets, yellow hornets, white-faced hornets and wasps (see also Chapter 6).

Rhinitis

It has become increasingly clear that immunotherapy with specific aeroallergen extracts is an effective treatment for allergic rhinitis, whether seasonal or perennial.

Asthma

The evidence for the effectiveness of immunotherapy for asthma caused by exposure to an aeroallergen is by no means as extensive as that for hay fever but, in general, it tells the same story. Ragweed, grass and birch pollen, cats, dogs, house dust mites and moulds have all been studied. The majority of controlled trials demonstrated beneficial effects of immunotherapy in both seasonal and perennial allergic asthma. However, despite continued use by specialists in allergy and immunology worldwide, immunotherapy for asthma is a perennial target for criticism by nonallergists who also care for patients with asthma.

Adverse reactions to foods

There have been no clinical studies indicating that food immunotherapy, either oral or by injection, has a role in the management of allergic individuals. One group of investigators demonstrated efficacy with immunotherapy in peanut-sensitive subjects, but many anaphylactic reactions occurred because of the allergen given.

Deciding when immunotherapy is appropriate

Hymenoptera venom anaphylaxis

The decision to use immunotherapy should be based on the severity of disease, the progression of symptoms, medication requirements, response to medication and the decrease in quality of life. Desensitization should be considered in people who have experienced a systemic reaction to an insect sting and who have positive puncture or intradermal skin tests to venom at a test concentration of 100 µg/ml or less. There are also special considerations regarding the risk of re-exposure (higher for beekeepers, gardeners, etc.), age (younger patients lose their sensitivity if not stung for a couple of years), the type of reaction (breathing difficulty and low blood pressure tend to reoccur), and the site of injection (laryngeal oedema can be fatal) (see Chapter 6).

Rhinitis and asthma due to aeroallergens

Both the severity and duration of allergy symptoms must be evaluated when considering immunotherapy. If the symptoms are moderately severe but of short duration, avoidance and pharmacotherapy should be tried first. When avoidance measures and medications are unsuccessful, immunotherapy may be appropriate. Perennial allergic rhinitis that responds poorly to medical therapy and avoidance may require immunotherapy. Patients who have tried both antihistamines and topical therapy and who have failed either because of lack of response or adverse effects may benefit from immunotherapy. Frequently, too little attention is paid to quality-of-life issues, such as the effect of allergic rhinitis on physical activity, intellectual performance, emotional interaction and social relationships. Poor performance at school and at work can clearly be traced to an intensification of these allergic conditions (***Table 10.1***).

Immunotherapy clearly requires a commitment of time and resources to be successful. Patients who cannot comply with medical pharmacotherapy and avoidance issues may find it difficult to comply with immunotherapy. Immunotherapy should be considered only in a setting where the ability to recognize and treat a systemic reaction is available.

The selection of appropriate antigens

Allergen selection

Allergens are selected for immunotherapy when exposure results in significant symptoms and when significant sensitivity has been demonstrated by skin tests or radioallergosorbent testing (RAST). This information should be combined with a thorough patient history with regard to the patient's environment and the timing of the symptoms. Allergens selected for immunotherapy should not be based on a positive skin or *in vitro* test alone.

The following antigens are considered effective for immunotherapy:

- grasses
- trees
- weeds
- mites
- animals (cats, dogs, horses)
- stinging insects (bees, wasps, yellowjackets, hornets).

When immunotherapy is considered, only standardized, high-potency extracts should be used. Extracts should contain all the pertinent, specific antigens identified. Over the years, standardization has continued to improve, resulting in

Table 10.1
Considerations for initiating immunotherapy.

Presence of IgE-mediated disease proven to benefit from immunotherapy
• Anaphylaxis following Hymenoptera stings.
• Allergic rhinitis.
• Allergic asthma.

Documentation of sensitivity to allergens associated with symptoms
• Suggestive personal history.
• There are positive skin test results or serum-specific IgE that correlates with symptoms.

Symptoms of sufficient duration and severity
• Anaphylaxis following Hymenoptera sting (except children with cutaneous anaphylaxis only).
• Two seasons of seasonal symptoms despite avoidance measures and pharmacologic therapy.
• Perennial symptoms, failing trials of avoidance measures and chronic pharmacologic therapy.

Availability of allergenic extract of allergen responsible for sensitivity

Other considerations
• Pharmacotherapy insufficiently controls symptoms or produces undesirable side-effects.
• Appropriate avoidance measures of indoor allergens fail to control symptoms.

• Discussion of long-term nature of treatment and need for compliance.
• Discussion of risk versus benefit of treatment.
• Accessibility of facilities and personnel capable of administering treatment and treating anaphylaxis.
• Emphasis of avoidance as treatment of choice.

The following conditions must be specifically evaluated before immunotherapy is considered:

• Concomitant therapy with a beta-blocker.
• Contraindication to the administration of adrenaline (epinephrine).
• Underlying ischaemic heart disease, cerebrovascular disease, severe chronic obstructive lung disease, uncontrolled hypertension, or those who are taking monoamine-oxidase inhibitors.
• Noncompliance by patients.
• Autoimmune disease (systemic lupus erythematosus, rheumatoid arthritis and other collagen vascular diseases).
• Induction but not maintenance therapy during pregnancy.
• Uncontrolled asthma.
• HIV status.
• Hypersensitivity conditions not exclusively dependent on IgE mechanisms (allergic bronchopulmonary aspergillosis and hypersensitivity pneumonitis).

higher-quality materials. The identification, preparation and standardization of allergenic extracts have changed through the years. Nonstandardized allergy extracts are defined by total protein content measured as protein nitrogen units (PNUs) or by weight and volume of diluent (W/V).

New standardization techniques are gradually being phased in. Manufacturers use a reference extract as a standard for comparison with the extracts they produce. WHO has approved methods for identifying, standardizing and storing allergenic extracts. The basic principles for standardization include the identification of the major allergens and a determination of their potency. The assignment of bioequivalent allergy units (BAUs) is based on a bioassay technique in selected patients highly allergic to a specific antigen. Using the Food and Drug Administration's (FDA) approved BAUs allows extracts to be compared no matter what their source. Other methods of standardization include allergy units (AUs), an *in vitro* assay and micrograms of the major antigens. *Table 10.2* lists some methods for comparing antigens.

Storage of allergen extracts

Allergen extracts should be maintained near labelled potency until used for diagnostic tests or immunotherapy. Because standard extracts lose their potency when stored at room temperature and with freezing and thawing, specific steps must be taken to preserve their potency. Allergen extracts should be kept at about 4 °C in a standard refrigerator. Dilutions of concentrated extracts lose their potency more rapidly than concentrated extract.

Table 10.2
Methods for comparing antigens.

Nonstandardized antigens
- Protein nitrogen unit (PNU)
- Weight by volume (W/V)

Standardized antigens
- BAU *in vivo* assay
- AU *in vitro* assay
- Micrograms of major antigens

Administering and monitoring (Table 10.3)

When specific immunotherapy (SIT) is indicated, a thorough discussion with the patient (including the potential dangers as well as the optimal duration of therapy) should be undertaken before the initiation of therapy. SIT should be prescribed by a specially trained physician and administered under the supervision of a physician trained to manage anaphylaxis. Adrenaline (epinephrine), corticosteroids and equipment for respiratory resuscitation must be readily available.

The starting dose is chosen so as to be well tolerated by even the most sensitive patient and the dose adjusted on the basis of patient history and skin testing results. Perennial immunotherapy begins with small incremental doses of allergens given once or twice a week. Allergy injections are given subcutaneously. The number of injections administered should be determined by the physician and should be based on the number of sensitivities. Increasing the number of allergens in a given vial of extract dilutes the amount of any single allergen delivered with each injection. This could jeopardize a beneficial response to treatment, as improvement is associated with larger amounts of each selected allergen administered. Allergen extracts are generally mixed in variable combinations as dictated by the pattern of patient sensitivity.

The gradual build-up to the maximum tolerated dose (called the *maintenance dose*) may vary from person to person based on the individual's sensitivities. The dose should be large enough to be effective and low enough to be safe. Generally, this is approximately 1 ml of the top concentration extract. Various schedules have been suggested for the administration of venom immunotherapy. Due to the unpredictability of life-threatening reactions to Hymenoptera stings, an accelerated immunotherapy schedule is often used. Using this accelerated schedule, and giving several injections each day, expedites the achievement of a maintenance dose for each venom employed. One hundred micrograms of each venom provides the equivalent of two or more natural stings. Some investigators have reported that 50 µg of each venom may be adequate. The maintenance dose is administered at 4–6 week intervals. If monthly maintenance doses of venom have been tolerated for 6 months, the interval between injections can be lengthened to 6–8 weeks or 8–12 weeks.

Table 10.3
Administering and monitoring immunotherapy.

Before the injection	Giving the injection	After the injection
• Patient's vials should be properly identified and expiry dates should be verified.	• Injections are given subcutaneously in the middle posterior third of the tricep using a 26- or 27-gauge needle.	• Patients should be observed in the office for 20–30 minutes after their injection, or longer if necessary, for any sign of anaphylaxis.
• Confirm the patient's first and last name and medical chart, and review the injection record.	• Aspirate before injecting the allergenic extract to be certain the needle has not entered a blood vessel. If so, the needle should be removed and new material administered in a different location.	• At the end of the waiting period, the injection site should be examined for a local reaction.
• Ask the patient about any delayed adverse reaction following his or her last immunotherapy injections. Identify any new problems or change in medication.		• Asthmatics may need to be auscultated.
• Pay special attention to the possible use of beta-blockers either as oral medication or as eye drops.		
• Asthmatic patients should be questioned carefully and auscultated for wheezing or other signs of asthma.	**Emergency equipment and supplies:**	
• Asthma patients need peak flow measurements before and after an allergy injection.	• stethoscope • sphygmomanometer • tourniquets, syringes • epinephrine (1:1000) • oxygen • intravenous fluids	
• Immunotherapy should not be administered if a patient is having breathing difficulties.	• oral airways • endotracheal tubes • antihistamines • corticosteroids • aminophylline • vasopressors • bronchodilator nebulizers	

The maintenance dose is usually administered at 2–4 week intervals provided the injections are well tolerated and symptoms improve. If systemic reactions or anaphylaxis occur, the physician should review the patient's immunotherapy history and adjust the dose of immunotherapy accordingly.

Adverse effects

Because the substance administered to the patient during immunotherapy has been proven to cause sensitivity to that patient, there is a risk that an adverse reaction may occur. The risk of significant adverse reactions is low, ranging from 0.05 to 3.5% per injection. Most of these adverse events are systemic manifestations of hypersensitivity, such as asthma, urticaria, laryngospasm, hypotension and angioedema. The majority of reactions occur during the build-up phase of treatment, and the patients who react are those with uncontrolled asthma.

Local reactions

Most patients receiving immunotherapy with extracts of aeroallergens will, at some time, have small areas of redness and swelling at the site of the injection that produce little discomfort and are of no concern. These reactions are to be distinguished from large local reactions 4 cm or greater in diameter that may cause considerable discomfort, may persist for 24 hours or longer and may be associated with a systemic reaction or may create concern that a further increase in dosage may cause a systemic reaction. Treatment consists of applying cold compresses, giving oral antihistamine and the reduction of the immunotherapy dose. Topical corticosteroid therapy or even systemic corticosteroid therapy may occasionally be necessary. There are no data to indicate that large local reactions are precursors of systemic anaphylactic reactions.

Vasovagal reactions

These must be differentiated from anaphylactic reactions. With vasovagal reactions, hypotension is associated with bradycardia rather than the tachycardia as seen in anaphylaxis. Cold or warm skin and perspiration may be present. There is no urticaria or angioedema. No medication is indicated for treatment. The patient usually responds promptly once in a recumbent position. No dose modifications are indicated.

Systemic reactions

The manifestations range in severity from a few hives to severe anaphylaxis and include the following systemic reactions:

- Flushing, sensation of warmth, diaphoresis.
- Urticaria: intense itching of palms, soles of feet or scalp.
- Fullness or 'lump' in throat.
- Chest tightness, wheezing, dyspnoea.
- Feeling of impending doom.
- Rhinitis, sneezing.
- Paroxysmal coughing, stridor, dysphonia.
- Nausea, vomiting, dizziness, fainting.
- Tachycardia, hypotension.
- Angioedema, conjunctivitis.
- Metallic taste in mouth.
- Uterine cramping.

Generally, urticaria or angioedema may occur. Swelling of the tongue, throat or lower airway can impair breathing and swallowing. Typical manifestations of hypovolemic shock may occur, including cold damp skin, rapid pulse and low blood pressure. Eye itching and tearing, nasal congestion and discharge, sneezing, coughing, wheezing and dyspnoea may occur. The reaction usually begins within 15 minutes of the injection. However, the reaction may be delayed from 30 minutes up to 6 hours after the injection. The cause of death in almost all subjects with asthma is respiratory, with or without anaphylactic shock. Neither the initial signs and symptoms of the systemic reaction nor a history of previous reactions to immunotherapy are predictive of fatality. *Table 10.4* outlines the circumstances under which systemic reactions may occur.

Injections should not be given if the patient has a fever or a flu-like illness or has unstable asthma or significant bronchospasm on the day of the injection. To decrease the likelihood of an anaphylactic reaction or limit the extent of anaphylaxis (should it occur), vigorous exercise should be avoided for 4 hours before and after an injection. The dose of maintenance immunotherapy during the major pollen season may be reduced. Because of the increased risk of anaphylaxis during the build-up phase, women should not begin a course of immunotherapy for allergic rhinitis while pregnant, although maintenance injections may be continued throughout pregnancy after discussing carefully the remote possibility of a systemic reaction and its risks to the foetus. Anaphylactic reactions should be treated promptly (see Chapter 5 for details) and the option of continuing immunotherapy should be carefully reviewed.

Table 10.4
Circumstances under which the frequency and severity of systemic reactions may increase.

1 Early months of immunotherapy when doses are being increased: **a** effective dose near highest tolerated dose; **b** large local reactions indicate need to reduce dose.
2 Errors in magnitude of dose: **a** patient incorrectly identified; **b** extract incorrectly identified; **c** dilution incorrectly identified; **d** dose incorrectly identified.
3 Intravenous administration of dose.
4 History of previous systemic reaction.
5 Patient highly sensitive.
6 Vigorous exercise just before/after injection.
7 New extract substituted.
8 Concomitant use of drugs that block beta-adrenergic receptors: **a** increased incidence of systemic reactions; **b** interference with treatment of systemic reactions with epinephrine; **c** interference with decisions about need for immunotherapy.
9 Presence of the start of a new illness or of fever.
10 Presence of uncontrolled asthma.
11 Natural exposure to a component allergen in the extract (e.g. grass pollen exposure in a patient receiving grass extract).

Adapted from Van Metre TE Jr. Immunotherapy for aeroallergen disease: circumstances under which the frequency and severity of systemic reactions may increase. In: Middleton E, Reed CE, Ellis EF et al. eds, *Allergy: Principles and Practice* (4th edn) (Mosby-Year Book Inc., St Louis, MO, 1993): 1501. Reproduced with permission.

If immunotherapy is being continued, the next dosage of the extract should be reduced by 2–4 steps and gradually escalated at weekly intervals until the maintenance dose is reached.
Retrospective studies of deaths following anaphylaxis associated with immunotherapy have indicated that patients with asthma are at higher risk of more severe anaphylactic reactions and fatal outcomes.

Evaluation of successful immunotherapy (Table 10.5)

It is important that the allergist regularly evaluates a patient during the first 18 months of immunotherapy. The allergist should look for improvement in symptoms, such as nasal congestion, rhinorrhoea, coughing, wheezing and secondary complications. The elimination or reduction of medications can follow effective immunotherapy. Objective measures, such as spirometry, nasal obstruction, snoring and mouth breathing, are also areas for consideration when evaluating the progress of effective immunotherapy.

Although subjective, improvement in the quality of life is important. Increased attendance and efficiency at school or work are important to the parent, teacher or employer as well as to the patient. There is no rationale for repeat skin testing to assess clinical effectiveness during immunotherapy, as skin tests may continue to be positive despite remission of symptoms. Repeat skin testing is helpful if the patient has developed new clinical sensitivities. Controlled sting challenges have been performed but they are not widely accepted.

Duration of venom immunotherapy

There is no consensus as to guidelines concerning the optimal duration of immunotherapy for Hymenoptera hypersensitivity. Various investigators have proposed and presented data supporting three approaches:

1 Measure the specific IgG to the venom used and discontinue immunotherapy when a concentration of 5 µg/ml or more is reached.
2 Repeat the measurement of specific IgE by either *in vitro* or skin testing and discontinue when the level decreases significantly from the initial value or disappears.
3 Discontinue without testing after immunotherapy has been given for a period of 3–5 years.

It is possible that all these approaches have clinical use. The application of clinical judgement plus the use of some of the aforementioned guidelines is generally the best course of action. Many studies suggest that venom immunotherapy can be discontinued after 3–5 years, irrespective of venom skin test results or venom-specific IgE or IgG levels. A five-year period of immunotherapy should be considered for people who have experienced:

Table 10.5
Patient assessment during immunotherapy.

• Symptom improvement.
• Medication reduction/elimination.
• Reduced school/work absenteeism.
• Improvement in quality of life.
• Improvement in secondary complications:
  – sinusitis
  – otitis media with effusion
  – nasal polyps
  – asthma.
	• Improvement in objective measures (spirometry, peak flow values, tympanometry, audiometry).
	• Sting challenges.

• severe anaphylactic shock before beginning immunotherapy;
• systemic reactions to venom immunotherapy injections.

Duration of aeroallergen immunotherapy

Data do not exist to identify the optimal duration of inhalant immunotherapy. Maintenance immunotherapy is usually administered until symptoms have improved to a satisfactory level for 1 year, until symptom improvement is noted in three consecutive annual seasons or, more preferably, 3–5 years of maintenance immunotherapy have been completed.

New methods

New directions in immunotherapy include the possibility of oral immunotherapy with selected allergens. The immunogenicity of immunotherapy using peptide fragments to activate T-cells that can modify the allergic response is being studied, and these products theoretically offer the benefits of conventional immunotherapy with a much reduced risk of systemic reactions to treatment. The manipulation of the allergic response using autologous immune complex therapy may be promising in the treatment of allergic rhinitis.

Local nasal areoallergen immunotherapy

Local nasal aeroallergen immunotherapy is an alternative form of immunotherapy using an aqueous solution of allergen to spray on the nasal mucosa at specified time intervals. The primary side-effects (pruritus, congestion and sneezing) are of sufficient severity in some subjects to result in discontinuation. Sufficient long-term trials are not yet available to permit a recommendation of this form of immunotherapy. Oral aeroallergen immunotherapy with birch pollen extract has been shown to be efficacious. A double-blind placebo-controlled trial of sublingual standardized cat immunotherapy for the treatment of asthma demonstrated no benefit. Oral immunotherapy is of uncertain efficacy, and additional studies are needed.

Alum-precipitated allergen extracts

Modification of aqueous extracts by precipitation of proteins with aluminium hydroxide results in a product that produces fewer systemic reactions than aqueous allergen extracts. This modification permits a more rapid increase in the dosage of the treatment, and fewer total injections are required before benefits are realized. Ragweed, cat and grass alum-precipitated extracts have

been studied and found to have the equivalent efficacy of aqueous extracts. Systemic reactions are decreased. Rarely, some patients experience a prolonged local reaction following the administration of alum-precipitated extracts. With alum-precipitated allergen extracts, subcutaneous nodules occur commonly at the sites of injections, but these are not troublesome and disappear soon if a different injection site is chosen.

Modified aeroallergen extracts

The aggregation of the proteins of an aqueous extract reduces the allergenicity while preserving the immunogenicity of the product. Two modifications have accomplished this: formalin-treated allergens (allergoids) and glutaraldehyde-treated allergens (polymerized allergen extracts). Regimens using these extracts permit completion of an immunotherapy programme with 10–15 injections, with a less than 1% occurrence of systemic reactions.

Peptide immunotherapy

In an attempt to circumvent systemic reactions related to IgE-induced mast cell degranulation, many allergens have been cloned and mutated to reduce interactions with IgE without changing the epitopes responsible for the development of T-cell tolerance. These peptides will inhibit Th_2 responses to allergens without triggering mast cell degranulation.

Vaccines

Mycobacteria have been shown to evoke IL-12 and consequently IFN-v production resulting in inhibition of Th_2 responses. One approach of treating allergy would be to take advantage of mycobacteria in modulating immune response towards a Th_1 type using the soil saprophyte, *M. vaccae*, since it is not a human pathogen. Clinical trials of this 'vaccine' for asthma and rhinitis are in progress with early results revealing efficacy.

The role of DNA vaccines in the management of allergic diseases is currently being studied. DNA encoding of a particular allergen could be incorporated into the genetic material of a plasmid or viral vector. Following administration into humans, this will replicate and induce endogenous production of allergenic proteins, which could subsequently activate T-cells.

Dendritic cells of vertebrates detect bacterial DNA through their excess of unprotected cytosine and guanosine nucleotide repeats (CpG). Synthetic DNA containing CpG motifs is recognised as a danger signal by receptors on dendritic cells, which serve to direct the T-lymphocyte response in a Th_1 type by inducing IL-12 release; this then enhances IFN-v production. Recent murine studies have shown that CpG DNA can be used alone or in conjunction with antigen to induce Th_1 response even in the presence of a pre-existing Th_2 response. Human studies in allergic rhinitis and asthma are being initiated using this strategy.

Immunotherapy has been tried for the treatment of food-induced allergic disorders. Using 'standard' immunotherapy in patients who experienced peanut-induced anaphylaxis, researchers have demonstrated that a minority of patients could tolerate larger quantities of peanuts for a prolonged period after rush therapy, but that the adverse reaction rate was unacceptable for standard clinical practice. On the other hand, immunotherapy with birch pollen has been effectively administered in patients with oral allergy syndrome.

Conclusion

Immunotherapy has been shown to be a

medically effective and cost-effective method for controlling allergic rhinitis and related diseases (such as allergic conjunctivitis, asthma and insect anaphylaxis) in those patients for whom pharmacotherapy does not prove effective and where avoidance is impossible or impractical. Careful and specific training is necessary for the physician to be able to conduct skin testing or *in vitro* testing to determine the allergens causing the reactions. Once these allergens are known and appropriate antigens prepared, immunotherapy must be carefully administered in a controlled and supervised environment where personnel are adequately trained to recognize and treat systemic reactions. It is best for the primary care physician who lacks training in immunotherapy to refer a patient whose symptoms indicate persistent allergy origins to an allergist with specialist training and knowledge in this field. The primary care physician, in consultation with the allergist, may then determine the appropriate course of treatment for that patient and work with the allergist to monitor the patient's progress.

Further reading

Fawcett WA IV. Allergy and immunology: allergen immunotherapy and avoidance. *Prim Care* (1998) **25:** 869–83.

Greineder DK. Risk management in asthma and allergic disease: risk management in allergen immunotherapy. *J Allergy Clin Immunol* (1996) **98:** 330–4.

Lehrer SB, Wild LG, Bost KL, Sorensen RU. Current knowledge and future directions: immunotherapy for food hypersensitivity. Food allergy. *Immunol Allergy Clin North Am* (1999) **19:** 563–81.

Nelson HS. Immunotherapy for inhalant allergens. In: Middleton E, Reed CE et al., eds. *Allergy: Principles and Practice* (5th edn) (Mosby-Year Book Inc., St Louis, MO, 1998).

Norman PS. Current reviews of allergy and clinical immunology: immunotherapy: past and present. *J Allergy Clin Immunol* (1998) **102:** 1–10.

Tippett J. Comprehensive care in the allergy/asthma office: allergen immunotherapy. *Immunol Allergy Clin North Am* (1999) **19:** 129–48.

WHO position paper. Allergen immunotherapy: therapeutic vaccines for allergic diseases. *Allergy* (1998) **53,** 44.

Latex allergy

11

Background

Hypersensitivity reactions to latex were first reported from Germany in 1927. The first report from the UK came in 1979 and since then this condition has been recognized worldwide. Between 1988 and 1992, the FDA received reports of more than 1000 systemic allergic reactions to latex, 15 of which were fatal. Although the true prevalence of latex allergy in the general population is not known it is widely believed that sensitization to this allergen has increased over recent decades, at least in the medical profession owing to the extensive use of latex gloves to avoid exposure to HIV and hepatitis infections. Those at risk of latex allergy include health care workers (5–30%), rubber industry workers (10%), patients with spina bifida (30–70%) and patients with other urogenital abnormalities. Data regarding the influence of age, gender, race and length of exposure to latex are inconsistent. However, it has been shown that atopic individuals are at a higher risk of developing allergy to latex than nonatopic individuals.

Latex allergen

Most natural rubber (99%) is derived from the latex (milky sap) of the commercial rubber tree, *Hevea brasiliensis*. The basic functional unit of latex is the spherical droplet (5 nm–3 µm) of polyisoprene which is coated with protein, lipid and phospholipid. One of the most important surface proteins that helps in polymerization of the basic units is prenyltransferase. Other important proteins in latex include hevein and hevamine. The antigenicity of latex has been characterized using immunochemical techniques and electrophoresis, and these are summarized in *Table 11.1*. Among more than 200 polypeptides present in natural rubber latex, about 60 were found to bind to IgE from sensitized patients.

Two major latex allergens have been identified: soluble hevein for latex-allergic health care workers and particle-bound rubber elongation factor (Hev b 1) for spina bifida patients. Ammonia or other preservatives (including sodium pentachlorophenate, tetramethylthiuram, sulphates, zinc oxide and sodium dimethyldithiocarbamate) are added to latex during the manufacturing process to prevent autocoagulation and bacterial contamination. Immunochemical studies have shown that nonammoniated latex extracts are better sources in which to study antigenicity than ammoniated extracts.

Clinical manifestation

Intolerance to latex can manifest itself in three forms:

- Irritant dermatitis.
- Type IV or delayed hypersensitivity reaction.
- Type I hyerpsensitivity reaction or latex allergy.

Irritant dermatitis, the most common reaction to latex, is caused by occlusion of the skin under the impermeable latex barrier. It results in dry, itchy, irritated areas, which may crack or break the skin. The second most common reaction is the delayed hypersensitivity type, and this is to the low molecular weight accelerators and antioxidants present in the rubber. The reaction occurs 1–2 days after contact, is limited to the area of contact and is erythematous, pruritic and sometimes results in blisters or vesciles. Diagnosis is confirmed by patch testing. These two reactions are not discussed

Table 11.1
The antigenicity of latex.

Antigen	Molecular weight	Remarks
Hev b1 or rubber elongation factor	14.6 kDa	Sensitization* in 50% of HCW and 80% of SB patients
Hev b 2 or β-1, 3-glucanase	36 kDa	
Hev b 3 or rubber particle protein	23 kDa	Allergenicity mainly restricted to SB patients
Hev b 4	50–57 kDa	Frequency of sensitization unknown
Hev b 5	25.6 kDa	Sensitization seen in 92% of HCW and 56% of SB patients. Hev b 5 exhibits high-sequence homology to an acidic protein from kiwi fruit
Hev b 6.01/6.02/6.03 (prohevein, hevein and prohevein C domain, respectively)	20 kDa	IgE reactivity is mainly due to hevein. Sensitization seen in 80% of latex-allergic HCW and 30% of SB patients
Hev b 7 or patatin-like allergen	46 kDa	Sensitization seen in 22.5% of latex-allergic HCW. These proteins are present in potatoes and tomatoes
Hevamine	29.5 kDa	Two basic isoforms A and B. Not an important allergen since sensitization is seen only in 3.4% of latex-allergic patients

* All sensitizations are expressed as a proportion of latex-allergic individuals.
HCW = health care workers; SB = spina bifida patients.

further in this chapter as the main focus is on latex allergy.

Type I reaction can manifest itself in several ways and in varying permutations and combinations in different individuals. Clinical manifestation depends at least in part on the route of exposure to the allergen. The most common form is contact urticaria appearing within 10–15 minutes after donning gloves. Redness, itching, wheal and flare response occur at the area of contact. Other reactions include rhinitis, conjunctivitis, wheezing, angioedema and anaphylaxis. Involvement of the upper and lower airways most commonly occurs following aerosolization of the allergen, especially following the use of powdered latex gloves. Serious life-threatening reactions, such as severe angioedema and anaphylaxis, have been reported following direct parenteral exposure or mucosal contact with latex gloves in an allergic individual during surgical procedures. Several reports have shown that latex allergy is often accompanied by sensitization to foods, such as bananas, avocados, apricots, grapes, passion fruit, pineapples, kiwi fruit, potatoes and chestnuts. In one study, 53% of 47 latex-allergic patients showed positive skin prick tests (SPTs) to avocados followed by potatoes (40%), bananas (38%), tomatoes (28%), chestnuts (28%) and kiwi fruit (28%). Interestingly, the majority of patients with positive SPTs did not show clinically relevant symptoms. This occurs because of the cross-reactivity between the allergens present in latex and these fruits and vegetables.

Investigation (Figure 11.1)

Diagnosis is often on clinical grounds. Although skin tests to latex are the gold standard in making a diagnosis of latex allergy, there is a small but real risk of provoking an anaphylactic reaction. Therefore, *in vitro* methods (enzyme-linked immunosorbent assays – ELISAs) are employed as a first step to detect circulating specific IgE to latex. In the presence of a good clinical history, a positive serum test is sufficient to make a diagnosis of latex allergy. In cases where the serum test is negative, SPTs should be performed. Latex extracts for SPTs are commercially available. Otherwise, fresh extracts can be prepared by washing and soaking a known quantity of the glove material in a known concentration of the diluent for varying lengths of time. In some centres, SPTs are carried out 'through' the latex glove.

It has to be borne in mind that the antigen content varies from glove to glove and

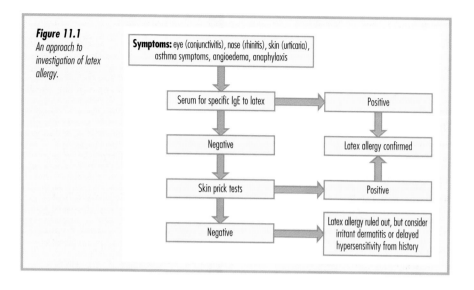

Figure 11.1
*An approach to
investigation of latex
allergy.*

Symptoms: eye (conjunctivitis), nose (rhinitis), skin (urticaria), asthma symptoms, angioedema, anaphylaxis

Serum for specific IgE to latex → Positive

Negative → Latex allergy confirmed

Skin prick tests → Positive

Negative → Latex allergy ruled out, but consider irritant dermatitis or delayed hypersensitivity from history

from brand to brand. It follows that it would be most reliable to skin test with the extract or glove from the same lot that caused the reaction. The sensitivity of SPTs can be increased through the use of two or more source materials. *Table 11.2* summarizes the sensitivity and specificity of skin tests versus ELISA in the diagnosis of latex allergy.

Management

At present, specific immunotherapy is not available for latex allergy. The key to the management of these patients is 'allergen avoidance', careful patient education and implementing appropriate changes in the work environment. In cases of latex-allergic patients undergoing invasive procedures, investigation or operations, the whole team should be alerted and special protocols of 'latex avoidance' should be implemented. These include the use of nonlatex gloves and materials during the procedures. In addition, such patients should be first on the list since it has been shown that the latex content of the operating environment is minimal at this time. Ideally, such patients should be

Table 11.2
Skin prick tests and serum tests in latex allergy.

	Sensitivity %	Specificity %	+ve predictive value	−ve predictive value
Skin prick tests	100*	99	80	100
Serum test	80–100**	63	?	98

* Sensitivity can be improved by using extracts from two or more sources.
** Depends on the kit and method employed.

operated on in special 'latex-free suites' but such facilities are not available in all hospitals.

As a preventive measure in patients with spina bifida and other urogenital abnormalities, it has been recommended that they should avoid exposure to latex from birth. In cases of health care workers allergic to latex, their colleagues should be alerted and only nonpowdered gloves should be used to prevent aerosolization of the antigen. Patients with latex allergy should also be provided with a medi-alert badge and an adrenaline auto-injector for emergency use.

Further reading

Avila PC, Shusterman DJ. Work-related asthma and latex allergy. *Postgrad Med* (1999) **105:** 39–46.

Posch A, Chen Z, Raulf-Heimsoth M, Baur X. Latex allergens. *Clin Exp Allergy* (1998) **28:** 134–40.

Ray B. Latex allergy: epidemic of the '90s. *Midwifery Today* (1998) Winter: 41–5.

Eosinophilic lung diseases

12

Introduction

Eosinophilic lung diseases are a heterogeneous group of disorders characterized by the presence of chest X-ray abnormalities and eosinophilia in the lung tissue with or without peripheral blood eosinophilia. The advent of fibreoptic bronchoscopy as an investigative tool and advances in molecular techniques have made it easier to study the airway lining fluid and alveolar tissue in patients with unexplained shadows on chest X-ray and to characterize the disorders and to understand their pathogenesis. *Table 12.1* lists the various clinical syndromes that present as pulmonary eosinophilia. There is a considerable overlap in the clinical presentation of these disorders but a careful clinical history and physical examination followed by detailed investigations often make it possible to arrive at the correct diagnosis. This chapter focuses mainly on the salient features of some of the commonly encountered eosinophilic lung diseases and on a clinical approach to patients with eosinophilic lung disease.

Table 12.1
Eosinophilic lung diseases.

Lung diseases commonly associated with eosinophilia:
- Simple pulmonary eosinophilia
- Chronic eosinophilic pneumonia (CEP)
- Acute eosinophilic pneumonia (AEP)
- Churg–Strauss syndrome (CSS)
- Asthma
- Allergic bronchopulmonary aspergillosis (ABPA)
- Bronchocentric granulomatosis
- Tropical pulmonary eosinophilia: filariasis, parasitic infections (*Ascaris, Ankylostoma, Schistosoma*)
- Drug reactions (*Table 12.4*)
- Idiopathic hypereosinophilic syndrome

Lung diseases sometimes associated with eosinophilia:
- Idiopathic pulmonary fibrosis
- Langerhan's cell granulomatosis
- Malignancies: small cell carcinomas, Hodgkin's disease, non-Hodgkin's lymphoma
- Fungal infections

In the following sections, some of the salient features of conditions leading to eosinophilic lung disease are discussed.

Simple pulmonary eosinophilia or Löffler's syndrome

This condition was first described by Löffler in 1932 and is characterized by migrating pulmonary infiltrates or shadows and peripheral blood (PBL) eosinophilia with minimal or no pulmonary symptoms. The chest X-ray often demonstrates a combined alveolar and interstitial pattern. Shadowing is usually subpleural, unilateral or bilateral, transient and fleeting. Most patients are eventually diagnosed as having a parasitic infection or a drug reaction but in over a third of patients no cause can be detected.

Treatment

First, rule out any underlying systemic disease. Withdraw the offending drug or treat the parasitic infection as the case may be. Cases of idiopathic type usually resolve spontaneously within a month and have an excellent prognosis.

Chronic eosinophilic pneumonia (CEP)

CEP usually occurs in the fifth decade of life and has a male:female ratio of 2:1.

Symptoms

CEP usually has an insidious onset and presents with cough, haemoptysis, fever, dyspnoea, weight loss and, occasionally, malaise, wheeze, cough with expectoration and night sweats. If constitutional symptoms predominate, pulmonary tuberculosis should be excluded. Interestingly, it has been reported that about half the patients with CEP have underlying asthma and in such patients ABPA should be considered in the differential diagnosis.

Investigations

Mild-to-moderate PBL and sputum eosinophilia, raised serum total IgE, ESR and thrombocytosis are usually seen. An increase in the titres of rheumatoid factor and immune complexes may also be noted.

Lung function tests

A restrictive pattern with a reduced carbon monoxide (CO) transfer factor is usually seen. The presence of any obstructive picture usually indicates underlying asthma.

Radiology

Peripheral lung infiltration is usually present. The classical appearance is of 'negative pulmonary oedema', i.e. dense, bilateral peripheral lung shadowing (also seen in bronchiolitis obliterans organizing pneumonia, sarcoidosis and drug reactions). Computed tomography (CT) scans allow better characterization.

Histopathology

Eosinophil and lymphocyte influx is seen in the interstitium and alveoli. Other features include interstitial fibrosis, bronchiolitis obliterans, eosinophil abscesses, low-grade vasculitis and noncaseating granulomas.

Bronchoalveolar lavage (BAL)

This usually demonstrates eosinophilia (>25%).

Treatment

Oral corticosteroids are the mainstay of treatment. Prednisolone in doses of 30–40 mg/d will produce dramatic resolution of symptoms within 1–2 days and radiographic abnormalities within 10 days. In order to prevent any relapse, prednisolone should be continued at a lower dose (5–20 mg) for 6 months.

Acute eosinophilic penumonia (AEP)

AEP is a disease of unknown aetiology and can present at any age. It usually starts as an acute febrile illness associated with myalgia, pleurisy and type I respiratory failure and often requires mechanical ventilation. Physical examination reveals fever, tachypnoea, expiratory rhonchi and basal crackles.

Investigations

Radiology
Chest X-rays and CT scans show diffuse parenchymal alveolar infiltrates involving all lobes, Kerley B lines and pleural effusions.

Lung function tests
These usually show a restrictive pattern with reduced CO diffusion capacity. PBL eosinophil counts and serum total IgE are normal. In contrast, BAL and pleural fluid show profound eosinophilia, together with a high pH suggesting degranulation of eosinophils.

Treatment
High-dose prednisolone is life saving in such patients. Methylprednisolone at a dose of 60–125 mg q.d.s is administered until the respiratory failure resolves. The dose can then be gradually tapered to 40–60 mg/d over the following 4–6 weeks. Typically, the disease does not relapse when corticosteroids are discontinued.

It is imperative to rule out *first* any infectious cause (viral, bacterial and fungal pneumonias) in such patients in view of the institution of high-dose steroid therapy. Early BAL should be performed if a diagnosis of AEP is suspected. Diagnosis should be suspected in patients with acute respiratory failure and who have unexplained pulmonary shadowing on chest X-ray.

Allergic bronchopulmonary aspergillosis (ABPA)

ABPA is a disorder resulting from an allergic response to inhaled fungal spores. In most instances it is *Aspergillus fumigatus* but could result from other fungal spores, including *Candida albicans, Aspergillus ochraceaus, A. oryzae, A. terreus, Curvularia lunata, Drechlera hawaiiensis, Geotrichum*

Figure 12.1 (a)
Chest X-ray PA view. A 57-year-old lady presented with worsening of her asthma symptoms, dyspnoea, cough, mucoid expectoration, malaise and weight loss. She had leucocytosis, peripheral blood eosinophilia, raised ESR and elevated serum total IgE. Chest X-ray shows evidence of bilateral non-segmental consolidation affecting one or two zones. Diagnosis: Allergic bronchopulmonary aspergillosis.

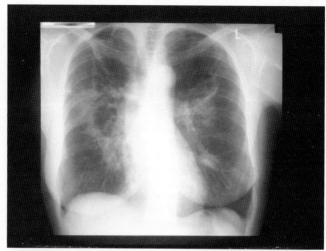

Figure 12.1 (b)
Chest X-ray PA view in the same patient after treatment with corticosteroids. Note the complete resolution of radiographic abnormalities.

Source: Radiographic film and legends provided by Dr D Delaney, Consultant Radiologist, Southampton General Hospital, Southampton, UK.

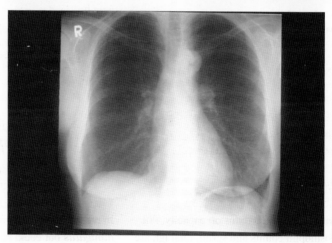

candidum, *Penicillium* and *Stemhylium lanuginosum*.

Clinical features

Most patients have underlying asthma. The disease presents in acute and chronic forms. Clinical symptoms are indistinguishable from asthma and the first clue to diagnosis is from the abnormalities seen on chest X-ray.

Serum total IgE is invariably raised. A normal serum total IgE virtually excludes the diagnosis. Skin prick tests (SPTs) to *Aspergillus fumigatus* are positive and the level of total IgE is markedly elevated and can be related to disease activity. *Aspergillus* precipitins are present in 90% of the patients when the serum is concentrated. In addition, there is marked PBL and BAL/sputum eosinophilia, and fungal hyphae can be detected in the sputum.

Radiology

Characteristically, ABPA affects the proximal airways of the upper lobes and causes 'central bronchiectasis'. Various chest X-ray patterns have been described in ABPA: 'gloved-finger appearance' when the bronchi are filled with secretions; 'tram line' sign when the medium-sized bronchi are inflamed and oedematous; and 'tooth paste' sign due to mucoid impaction in the bronchus and consolidation secondary to airway obstruction.

Treatment

The successful treatment of ABPA centres around the eradication of the fungal spores from the airways, adequate control of asthma symptoms, effective physiotherapy to dislodge any mucus plugs from the airways and the prevention of the irreversible fibrotic process. In the acute stage, prednisolone should be given at a dose of 40–60 mg/d until there is complete resolution of symptoms and clearance of radiological abnormalities. Steroid dosage could then be tapered and finally discontinued. Any mucus plug impaction in the airways that is not cleared with steroids and physiotherapy can be removed by fibreoptic bronchoscopy.

In the chronic stage, patients should be kept at the lowest dose of steroids, together with bronchodilators if necessary to control their symptoms. Follow-ups of patients in case studies have shown that long-term corticosteroids may prevent progress to end-stage fibrosis. Two important unresolved issues in the management of patients with ABPA are

1 whether patients should receive maintenance corticosteroids in remission or only those patients with recurrent exacerbations; and 2 the role of antifungal drugs.

Idiopathic hypereosinophilic syndrome (HES)

HES is a multisystem disorder characterized by PBL eosinophilia together with a marked influx of eosinophils into several organs that causes damage. The disorder is associated with a clonal expansion of the CD4 T-cell subset, suggesting a link. Immature cells of eosinophilic lineage may be seen in peripheral blood. It is usually seen in the third or fourth decade of life and has a male preponderance (7:1).

Clinical picture

Systemic constitutional symptoms including night sweats, weight loss, pruritis, anorexia, fever and organ-associated symptoms (usually pulmonary and cardiac). Cardiac involvement usually causes endomyocardial fibrosis resulting in restrictive cardiomyopathy. Mural thrombosis and thromboembolism (deep vein thrombosis and pulmonary embolism) are the major causes of morbidity and mortality. Pulmonary involvement leads to infiltration, pleural effusions and fibrosis. Nervous system involvement may result in stroke, peripheral neuropathy and mononeuritis multiplex. Other organs involved include the peripheral nerves, the gastrointestinal tract, the skin, muscles, joints and kidneys.

Treatment

High-dose corticosteroids (prednisolone 60 mg/d) will result in the resolution of symptoms in 50% of patients. Corticosteroids may have to be continued for over 3 months and then gradually tapered, depending on the clinical response. Patients with a history of thromboembolism would need long-term anticoagulation with warfarin. Immunosuppressive agents including busulphan, hydroxyurea, cyclophosphamide, azathioprine, interferon-α, cyclosporine-A, etoposide and vincristine have been used with success.

Churg–Strauss syndrome/allergic angiitis or granulomatosis

Churg–Strauss syndrome (CSS) is a systemic disorder of unknown aetiology. It presents as an allergic airways disease (such as asthma or allergic rhinitis) for at least 8–10 years before the full-blown syndrome becomes apparent. This is followed by the appearance of PBL eosinophilia and the influx of various organs with eosinophils. The third phase is full-blown systemic vasculitis but this is not frequently seen since most patients are already on corticosteroid therapy by that time. The various clinical manifestations of this condition are summarized in *Table 12.2*.

Investigations

Radiology

Patchy transient infiltrates, nodules, diffuse interstitial infiltrates and pleural effusions can occur. Hepatic and renal angiograms may demonstrate aneurysms resembling those in polyarteritis nodosa.

BAL and PBL eosinophilia are common. Serum total IgE is elevated and correlates with disease activity. Normochromic normocytic anaemia, raised ESR,

Table 12.2
The clinical features of Churg–Strauss syndrome.

System	Symptoms
Cardiovascular system	Hypertension, angina, pericarditis, heart failure, arrhythmias, sudden death
Respiratory system	Sinusitis, rhinitis, nasal polyps, asthma
Gastrointestinal tract	Abdominal pain, diarrhoea, gastrointestinal bleed
Skin	Nodules, purpura, vasculitis
Kidney	Renal insufficiency, nephrotic syndrome, focal segmental glomerulonephritis
Joints	Arthralgia
Neurological system	Mononeuritis multiplex, peripheral neuropathy, cerebral haemorrhage
General	Fever, myalgia

rheumatoid factor and reduced serum complement levels are other associated, but nonspecific, features.

Antineutrophil cytoplasmic antibody (ANCA)

Some 50% of patients with this syndrome have a perinuclear (p)-ANCA. This is a useful marker to differentiate the condition from Wegener's granulomatosis, which is characterized by the presence of cytoplasmic (c)-ANCA.

Open lung biopsy

The main findings include necrotizing vasculitis, interstitial and perivascular granulomas and tissue eosinophilia.

Treatment

As in the other conditions described above, corticosteroids are the mainstay of treatment. Prednisolone at a dose of 0.5–1.0 mg/kg/day is required for several weeks until the vasculitis resolves fully. This should be followed by low-dose maintenance therapy for at least a year. When extremely high doses of corticosteroids are required to suppress disease activity, steroid-sparing agents such as cyclophosphamide or azathioprine are used.

Tropical pulmonary eosinophilia (TE) and parasitic infections

TE results from a hypersensitivity response to the presence of a microfilarial parasite (including *Wuchereria bancrofti* or *Brugia malayi*) in the lymphatic system. It is a common condition frequently misdiagnosed as bronchial asthma in India, Sri Lanka, China, Africa and southeast Asia, where this disorder is most common. It is more common in people visiting endemic areas from a nonendemic area than in people resident in an endemic area. Not surprisingly, the diagnosis of this condition requires a high index of clinical suspicion, particularly in western countries where it is extremely rare.

Clinical features: a dry cough, breathlessness and wheeze.

Investigations

Investigations should establish a PBL/BAL eosinophilia of $\geq 3000/mm^3$, a markedly raised serum total IgE ≥ 1000 U/ml, the *absence* of a microfilarial parasite in concentrated blood samples collected during the night and day, leucocytosis and raised ESR.

Serology

High titres of antifilarial IgE and IgG are detectable (these can cross-react with other helminthic Ags, so caution should be exercised in interpretation).

Lung function tests

There is predominantly an obstructive defect but a mixed picture might be present in chronic cases. Bronchial hyper-responsiveness with reversible airway obstruction may also be present.

Radiology

Reticulonodular opacities, miliary mottling, prominent hila and increased bronchovascular markings have been reported, mainly affecting the mid and lower zones on chest X-ray.

Treatment

Diethylcarbamazine (DEC) is the drug of choice (6 mg/kg for 3 weeks is the recommended dose). Patients with TE respond favourably to treatment and this can be used as a reliable criterion for diagnosis. Some 20% of patients relapse and, in such cases, a higher dose of 12 mg/kg can be given for another 3–4 weeks. Early and effective treatment can prevent pulmonary fibrosis and chronic respiratory failure.

Parasitic infections

Parasitic infections are a common cause of pulmonary eosinophilia in the developing world. A number of parasites pass through the human lung during their life-cycles and, during passage, trigger a hypersensitivity reaction resulting in pulmonary eosinophilia. The parasites that cause pulmonary eosinophilia are listed in **Table 12.3**. Clinical features include skin rashes, a dry cough, breathlessness, wheeze and, rarely, chest pains and haemoptysis can occur. Peripheral blood and BAL eosinophilia, raised serum total IgE, pulmonary infiltrates and a restrictive pattern of lung function are seen in most cases. Auscultation may reveal crackles and rhonchi. Stool examination is usually negative because the pulmonary phase precedes the development of the larvae into adult worms in the intestines in most cases. It follows that a high index of clinical suspicion is essential to make a diagnosis. Specific treatment with antihelminthic drugs should be instituted as early as possible. In severe cases, a short course of corticosteroids is beneficial.

Table 12.3
Parasites that cause pulmonary eosinophilia.

NEMATODES
Ankylostoma sp (hook worm)
Ascaris sp (round worm)
Strongyloides stercolaris
Trichinella spiralis (dog round worm)
Toxocara

Filariasis:
Wuchereria bancrofti (filarial parasite)
Brugia malayi (filarial parasite)
Dirofilaria immitis

TREMATODES
Paragonimus westermani (lung fluke)
Schistosoma

CESTODES
Echinococcus sp (hydatid)

Drug reactions

Drugs are one of the commonest causes of pulmonary eosinophilia seen in clinical practice. Reactions can lead to PBL/BAL eosinophilia and pulmonary infiltrates. Some of the drugs reported to cause these disorders are listed in **Table 12.4**. Prompt withdrawal of the drug is mandatory and, in severe cases, a short course of prednisolone will hasten the recovery process.

There are a few other disorders listed in **Table 12.1** that could lead to pulmonary eosinophilia but these are not discussed in this chapter.

A clinical approach to the patient with eosinophilic lung disease

The following section together with **Figure 12.2** summarizes a broad clinical approach in a patient with pulmonary eosinophilia.

Table 12.4
Drugs that can cause pulmonary eosinophilia.

- **Antibiotics:** ampicillin, minocycline, nitrofurantoin, penicillin, tetracycline, sulphonamides
- **NSAIDs:** diclofenac, naproxen, fenbrufen, ibuprofen, para-amino salicylic acid, piroxicam, tolfenamic acid, loxoprofen
- **Antiasthma drugs:** beclomethasone dipropionate, disodium cromoglycate, leukotriene receptor antagonists (montelukast, zafirlukast)
- **Cytotoxic drugs:** bleomycin, methotrexate
- **Antiepileptics:** carbamazepine, phenytoin, valproic acid
- Chlorpromazine
- **Cytokines:** GM-CSF, IL-2, IL-3
- Sulphasalazine
- **Antimalarial:** Fansidar (sulphadoxine + pyrimethamine)
- Clofibrate
- L-tryptophan
- Rapeseed oil
- Acetaminophen
- Cocaine
- **Angiotensin converting enzyme inhibitors:** captopril, enalapril, fosinopril
- **5-hydroxytryptamine and noradrenaline reuptake inhibitors:** venlafaxine

---

History

- Acute or chronic presentation.
- Enquire about associated systemic or organ-based symptoms for connective tissue disorders and malignancy.
- Any exposure to drugs that can induce pulmonary eosinophilia.
- Risk for HIV infection.
- Travel history for filariasis and parasitic infection.
- History of allergic rhinitis and asthma: associated with Churg–Strauss syndrome, ABPA, bronchocentric granulomatosis.
- Contact with animals (Toxocara, hydatid disease).

Investigations

(a) Peripheral blood eosinophilia:
   - Present: tropical pulmonary

Figure 12.2
A systemic clinical approach to a patient with pulmonary eosinophilia.

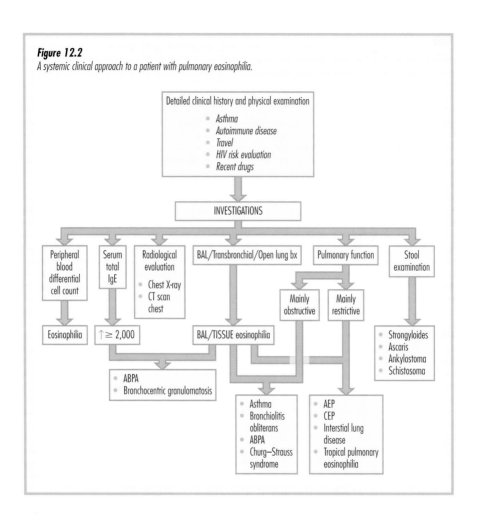

eosinophilia, CEP, simple
pulmonary eosinophilia, ABPA,
hypereosinophilic syndrome.
- Absent: AEP, PCP and drug
reactions.

(b) Stool and serological examination for
parasites.

(c) Serum total IgE, ESR and C-reactive
proteins.

(d) SPT and precipitins for aspergillus.

(e) Pulmonary function tests, including
spirometry and gas transfer factor.

(f) Chest X-ray, CT scan of chest.

(g) Fibreoptic bronchoscopy for BAL
fluid (eosinophilia and for bacteria
and fungi) and transbronchial
biopsies.

(h) Open lung biopsy if needed.

Acknowledgements

The authors are grateful to Dr R Limbrey
for providing some useful information on
ABPA.

Further reading

Allen JN, Bruce-Davis W. Eosinophilic
lung diseases. *Am J Respir Crit Care Med*
(1994) **150:** 1423–38.

Extrinsic allergic alveolitis

13

Introduction

Extrinsic allergic alveolitis (EAA) (or hypersensitivity pneumonitis) are a group of disorders characterized by granulomatous inflammation affecting the peripheral gas-exchanging portions of the lung in response to repeated inhalation of organic dusts. The organic dusts implicated in this condition can be broadly categorized into two major groups:

- Microbial spores growing on vegetable matter (such as hay, straw, mushroom compost, sugarcane, etc.).
- Avian (from pigeons, budgerigars, parrots, turkeys) and mammalian proteins (bovine and pituitary extracts).

In addition, some cases of EAA have been reported in response to isocyanates and drugs.

EAA is mainly an occupational disease predominantly affecting farmers (farmer's lung) and those who come into close contact with birds (bird fancier's lung) – such as those who breed and keep pigeons for racing. EAA was first described by Campbell as farmer's lung in 1932. Since then there have been several reports of EAA and the condition has now been well characterized. In bird fancier's lung, a glycoprotein antigen present in the excreta of birds and in the bloom of their feathers is disseminated into the environment and this can be inhaled by people coming into close contact with it. This triggers of a granulomatous reaction in some individuals. The main antigens implicated in farmer's lung are *Micropolyspora faeni* and the *Thermophilic Actinomycetes* spp. *T. vulgaris* and *T. sacchari*. Several other causes of EAA have been identified and some of these are summarized in *Table 13.1*.

Table 13.1
Common causes of EAA.

Disease	Source/*antigen*
Farmer's lung	Mouldy hay, compost, straw; *M. faeni*
Bird fancier's lung	Bird bloom; *avian proteins*
Bagassosis	Mouldy bagasse; *T. sacchari*
Mushroom worker's lung	Spores, mouldy compost; *M. faeni*
Cheese worker's lung	Cheese mould; *Penicillium caseii*
Ventilation pneumonitis	Contaminated air conditioners; *Acanthamoeba castellani, Naeglaria gruberi*
Malt worker's lung	Mouldy malt; *Aspergillus*
Coffee worker's lung	Coffee beans; *coffee bean dust*
Compost worker's lung	Compost; *Aspergillus spp.*
Detergent worker's lung	Detergent; *Bacillus subtilis enzymes*
Ventilation pneumonitis	Contaminated water in air conditioners; *Aureobasidium pullulans*
Japanese summer house pneumonitis	House dust, bird droppings; *Trichosporon cutaneum*
Tobacco worker's lung	Mould on tobacco; *Aspergillus spp.*
Wood worker's lung	Dust from wood; *Alternaria*
Spray-paint worker's lung	Isocyanates

It appears likely that between 5 and 15% of an exposed population will develop EAA and that the immunogenicity of the organic dust, the exposure level and host factors are important determinants in the development of the disease. The prevalence of EAA has mainly been studied in certain occupational groups (such as farmers or bird breeders) and the published figures have been variable, depending upon the criteria used to define the disease. Questionnaire surveys have shown higher prevalence rates than studies that took into account the presence of serum precipitins, since a detectable antibody is present in only 50% of patients who have the condition. There are over 80 000 registered pigeon fanciers in the UK, and a further 12% of the population have budgerigars in their homes. Around 5% of pigeon fanciers and 1–2% of budgerigar keepers develop alveolitis. It is estimated that 1 in 1000 of the population has bird fanciers's lung to some degree. Amongst farm workers in England and Wales, EAA affects 117 per 1000 and 129 per 1000, respectively. When serology was taken into account, the figures fell to 22 and 54 per 1000, respectively. The prevalence rate in Wisconsin farm workers, where much more stringent criteria were used was 4.2 per 1000. The incidence of occupationally related alveolitis in the UK (SWORD Scheme) between 1991 and 1997 have been mainly related to farming (54%), birds (34%), mushroom workers (12%), humidifiers (12%). The remaining cases which constituted relatively minor proportions were mainly related to marine proteins, isocyanates, rubber, chemicals and metals.

Pathology and pathogenesis

Although classified as an allergic alveolitis, EAA does not result from a type I hypersensitivity reaction. It has been described as a type III hypersensitivity reaction involving the deposition of immune complexes and the activation of complement. The classical description of the lesion in EAA is the presence of bronchocentric noncaseating granulomas with plasma cells, lymphocytes, macrophages, epitheloid and giant cells. The granulomas tend to occlude the bronchioli and alveoli. The bronchocentric nature of inflammation, together with interstitial involvement, distinguish it from a sarcoid granuloma. In the chronic state, the granulomas lead to fibrosis that predominantly affects the upper lobes.

The pathogenesis of EAA is not fully understood and is beyond the scope of this book. Several different hypotheses have been put forward. Early views supported the role of IgG antibodies and the deposition of immune complexes in the peripheral airways followed by the activation of complement. Subsequent studies have proven that there is a poor correlation between serum precipitins and disease activity. Recent bronchoalveolar lavage (BAL) studies have shown some interesting abnormalities in T-cell subsets, supporting the role of T-cells in the disease process.

Lymphocytosis in BAL fluid, as in sarcoidosis, has been described both in asymptomatic as well as symptomatic patients. Whilst the CD4:CD8 ratio increases to 5:1 in sarcoidosis, in EAA the ratio is normal or <1 due to relative CD8 lymphocytosis. It has been suggested that suppression of the disease is mediated by suppressor T lymphocytes and, in symptomatic patients, there may be a breakdown in immune regulation, leading to these cells becoming nonfunctional. Consistent with this view, abnormal activation of CD8+ve lymphocytes in response to antigenic stimulation has been described in symptomatic patients. Markers of activation, such as HLA-DR and mixed lymphocyte response (MLR) 1–3, have been identified on lymphocytes in BAL fluid from symptomatic patients with EAA.

Clinical features

EAA has been described in acute, subacute and chronic forms. In the classic form of acute EAA, symptoms become apparent 6–8 hours after antigenic exposure and include breathlessness, cough, fever, malaise, myalgia and headache. If there is no further antigenic exposure, symptoms resolve within 48 hours but sometimes can take longer (up to a week). In cases of recurrent exposure, symptoms can become unremitting and more severe, which is sometimes described as the subacute form of the illness. The subacute form is more likely to present as an insidious onset of breathlessness and cough over a few weeks.

If there is continued antigenic exposure, fibrotic changes begin to appear in the lungs and these could lead to chronic irreversible lung damage. In some cases patients come into medical attention for the first time after irreversible changes have occurred but who have no previous history of acute/subacute EAA. This could be because low levels of continued antigenic exposure are not sufficient to promote an acute episode, but the cumulative exposure leads to fibrosis and loss of respiratory reserve.

Clinical examination during an acute episode may reveal inspiratory crackles or 'squeaks' from obstructed peripheral airways. Sometimes clinical examination may be unremarkable. In chronic forms, digital clubbing is present in 50% of cases and examination will usually reveal inspiratory crackles due to underlying fibrosis.

Diagnosis of EAA is made from a combination of positive findings from a careful clinical/occupational history, a clinical examination and serological and radiological evidence. In doubtful cases a bronchial inhalation challenge can be performed. A fall in forced vital capacity (FVC), an increase in body temperature and peripheral blood neutrophilia are reliable markers to distinguish 'responders' from 'nonresponders'. Other characteristic abnormalities in an acute reaction are hyperventilation, restriction of ventilation, a decrease in TLCO and hypoxaemia. The investigations used in EAA are summarized in *Table 13.2*.

EAA should be differentiated from certain other conditions, and these are summarized in *Table 13.3*.

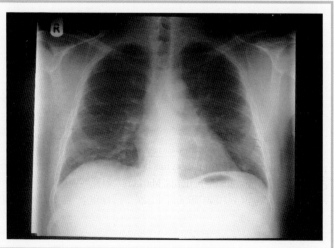

Figure 13.1 (a)
Chest X-ray PA view. A 43-year-old man presented with shortness of breath. Chest X-ray shows decrease in lung volumes together with ground glass appearance.

Source: Radiographic film and legend provided by Dr D Delaney, Consultant Radiologist, Southampton General Hospital, Southampton, UK.

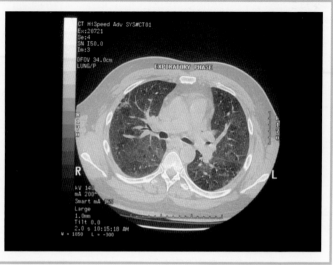

Figure 13.1 (b)
CT scan of chest from the same patient. Note the geographical ground glass appearance of the parenchyma. Diagnosis: Extrinsic allergic alveolitis. (He had a parakeet in his bedroom)

Source: Radiographic film and legend provided by Dr D Delaney, Consultant Radiologist, Southampton General Hospital, Southampton, UK.

Management

Patient education and counselling are of the utmost importance in long-term management. Patients should be advised about the risk of continued exposure and irreversible lung changes. Most patients are unhappy to change their occupation since this will completely change their lifestyles and livelihoods, and this may have huge financial implications for their families. Hence methods to improve the working environment to reduce the level of antigenic exposure are essential.

Wearing pollen masks, personal dust respirators, air stream helmets and ventilated helmets is a highly efficient way of purifying the air. Other measures including keeping crops dry and well ventilated during storage to reduce the growth of thermophilic organisms, the addition of 1% propionic acid to prevent moulding in stored grains and, in the case of bird breeders, careful loft design, careful handling of bird excreta and the wearing of protective clothes.

Most patients with acute illness recover well with bed rest and removal from the

Table 13.2
Investigations into EAA.

Investigation	Findings	Comments
FBC CRP, ESR IgE Other Igs Chest X-ray	Leucocytosis, mild eosinophilia ↑ Normal Small increase in IgG and M **Acute:** normal or: • ground glass infiltration • loss of sharpness of blood vessels • nodular or micronodular lesions • patchy consolidation **Chronic:** • linear shadowing • honey combing • loss of volume, mainly in upper lobes	Acute EAA
CT scan	**Acute:** patchy or diffuse ground glass infiltration or nodular shadowing **Chronic:** loss of architecture, linear shadowing, shrinkage and fibrotic changes	Can be seen when chest X-ray is normal No calcification seen
PFTs	↓ in VC, TLC, RV FEV_1/FVC: normal or ↑ TLCO: ↓	Restrictive pattern
Serum precipitins to causative organisms	Mainly IgG, sometimes Ig A and M	Greater sensitivity than specificity in acute illness. Up to 15% of subjects with current exposure but asymptomatic will have detectable precipitins

Table 13.3
Differential diagnosis.

Differential diagnosis	Comments
Atypical and other pneumonias	Due to mycoplasma, legionella, viruses, PCP, miliary TB
Fibrosing alveolitis	Clubbing, late inspiratory crackles
Acute pulmonary drug reactions (nitrofurantoin, penicillins, sulphonamides)	History + PBL eosinophilia
Silofiller's lung	Due to exposure to oxides of nitrogen from fresh silage. Usually affects several people exposed at the same time. Chest X-ray shows noncardiogenic pulmonary oedema
Pulmonary mycotoxicosis	From inhalation of organic dust during removal of top layer of silage. Acute febrile illness after a few hours of exposure without chest X-ray changes
Sarcoidosis	Other clinical features: erythema nodosum, uveitis, skin involvement, hilar adenopathy, BAL fluid shows ↑ CD4:CD8
Allergic bronchopulmonary aspergillosis	Usually underlying asthma; affects upper lobes; central/perihilar distribution; SPT/RAST positive to *Aspergillus fumigatus*; radiological signs help to differentiate
Chronic beryllium disease	Occupational history; beryllium lymphocyte transformation test is characteristically positive

environment. Sometimes acute or subacute illness may be severe enough to warrant hospitalization and supportive treatment with oxygen, bronchodilators and oral corticosteroids. Several studies have shown that oral steroids help speedy recovery during an acute illness but do not seem to have any effect on long-term prognosis. Prednisolone is given at a dose of 1 mg/kg for 1–2 weeks and tapered thereafter over the following 2–4 weeks. Some authors recommend a trial dose of prednisolone, even in the chronic stage.

If the patient decides to return to his or her occupation, he or she should be followed up periodically with serological, physiological and radiological investigations. Any worsening of clinical symptoms, lung function or radiological parameters warrants immediate removal of the patient from the working environment to avoid any further exposure.

Further reading

Daroowalla F, Raghu G. Hypersensitivity pneumonitis. *Comprehensive Therapy* (1997) **23:** 244–8.

Reynolds SP. Extrinsic allergic alveolitis: an easily overlooked diagnosis. *Br J Hosp Med* (1994) **52:** 257–9.

Index